NO FAULT WITH NO FEAR

A Chiropractor's Guide to Ethical and Clinical Excellence in Personal Injury Practice

S. Joseph Metz, DC

Copyright © 2017 S. Joseph Metz

No portion of this book may be reproduced in any form without written permission.

All rights reserved.

Cover concept by S. Joseph Metz

Author Contact:
drfeelgood35@hotmail.com

ISBN: 1977640958
ISBN-13: 978-1977640956

To Sandy

and

To Joely

TABLE OF CONTENTS

	Acknowledgments	9
	Introduction	13
1	The No-Fault Industry	19
2	Clinics: The Lay of the Land	29
3	Fraud and its Forms	51
4	Insurance Industry Response	73
5	Legal Ramifications	79
6	Case Studies in Fraud	89
7	Excellence in the Clinic	109
8	Patient Intake	113
9	Initial Interview & History	119
10	Examination	125
11	Imaging	145
12	Other Testing	153
13	Diagnosis & Treatment	157
14	Recordkeeping	177
15	Discharge	185
16	Working for a Living	193

Afterword	205
Appendix A- No-Fault Law	209
Appendix B- Clinical Forms	225
Appendix C- No-Fault Forms	233
Appendix D- Common Diagnosis Codes	241

NO-FAULT WITH NO FEAR

ACKNOWLEDGMENTS

They say it takes a village to raise a child, and in the sense that writing a book has been likened to a kind of birthing process, the saying applies here as well. A small village's worth of people was gracious enough to help with this book, and raise this "child": Shlomit Metz-Poolat, Esq., checked and corrected me on the criminal legal stuff; Avi Meir, Esq., set me straight on some of the no-fault technicalities; and Marc Weber, MD reviewed the clinical section to make sure I didn't mess anything up too terribly. Martin Bluth, MD, PhD gave me valuable feedback. Tami Schwartz and Tom Galitsis graciously lent their considerable editing skills and advice toward cleaning up the manuscript. Steve Agocs, DC, Associate Professor at Cleveland University-Kansas City helped with verifying chiropractic historical data. They are all experts in their respective professions, so any errors you may come across are mine alone.

NO FAULT WITH NO FEAR

INTRODUCTION

The alternative title of this book could be *How To Practice No-Fault Without Getting Into Legal, Ethical, or Clinical Trouble*. It's probably safe to assume that most Doctors of Chiropractic in New York, at least in the downstate region, practice within the no-fault environment (known as "doing no-fault") at least to some degree. Recent decades have seen a proliferation of multidisciplinary clinics where virtually 100% of the patient cases are no-fault. Especially if you don't own your own practice, and need to work for a living, there's at least a 50 percent chance that you'll be working in a no-fault clinic (see Chapter 5), and in the New York metropolitan area, no-fault probably sustains the vast majority of chiropractors' practices. It is, for better or for worse, the most reliable type of case for generating consistent revenue. Accidents will always happen; injuries take time to heal and require frequent and regular patient visits. Patients are often involved in litigation, which helps motivate them to keep coming in. In fact, I would go as far as to say that if tomorrow, chiropractic was no longer covered under no-fault benefits in New York, half the profession would vanish overnight.

Unfortunately, no-fault practice has something of a sleazy reputation, and it's not entirely undeserved. Fraud is prevalent throughout the industry, and not just among chiropractors, but unfortunately, chiropractors are involved too often. There have been too many news stories about takedowns of crooked no-fault rings that include the arrest of chiropractors. Recent years have seen a crackdown on fraud involving no-fault, with arrests and convictions of both medical and chiropractic doctors, acupuncturists, office managers, clinic owners, and others. In nearly twenty-five years of practice in the New York metropolitan area, I have worked as both an employee (associate) doctor and as a cover/per diem doctor in dozens of dedicated no-fault clinics, as well as owned a private practice that included no-fault in the patient mix. I've seen the good, bad, and plain ugly aspects of the no-fault industry, and some of the chiropractors who operate within it.

This book confronts issues germane to the practice of personal injury chiropractic mainly in New York, especially in the New York City metropolitan area, though other states (like Minnesota and Michigan) have similar no-fault systems, and similar issues. It's also written with a mind toward newer practitioners—it's the book I wish I had been able to read when I began practice as a new graduate. However, more experienced doctors will also find it useful, and a good part of the information in these pages, such as the clinical section, is certainly applicable to other locales and to the practice of chiropractic in general.

What this book is not: It's not a book on how to "play" the no-fault system. It won't teach you how to get more patients or make more money. I don't have any secret practice "system." All I have is experience and information to share with you that I mostly accumulated the hard way, and that I hope you can learn from. What I hope this book will accomplish is to help you practice chiropractic as safely and ethically as possible within the no-fault system. I hope it will help you be a better doctor, and give you better insight into what to watch out for when working in the field.

You might read this book and think that the information and advice in it should be obvious. Sadly, I'm here to tell you it isn't—or, at any rate, too many doctors aren't heeding it. If you're the kind of doctor who thinks there's nothing this book can teach you, you might be exactly the kind of doctor who needs to read it. I learned quite a bit while researching this book, and if there were things I didn't know after almost 25 years of practice, chances are you might learn something too.

I've been in love with chiropractic ever since I was a teenager, when I first became a patient. Like many love affairs, it hasn't always been smooth or easy; I've had my heart broken, and I've made more than my share of mistakes along the way. But I believe that chiropractic has a special place among the healing professions, and that even—especially—in the personal injury domain, we can shine. This book is my attempt to help our profession strive towards ethical and professional excellence, so that both new and more experienced doctors are more aware of potential legal and clinical pitfalls, and most importantly, so that no chiropractor's name appears in a news article about fraud ever again.

S. Joseph Metz, DC

NO-FAULT WITH NO FEAR

I
INCIDENTS AND ACCIDENTS

"They're funny things, accidents. You never have them till you're having them."
—A. A. Milne

1

THE NO-FAULT INDUSTRY

Driving is dangerous. Whether you live and drive in the city, a suburb, or a rural area—and I've lived and driven in all three—operating a motor vehicle always carries with it a certain degree of risk. Weather conditions, traffic, other drivers, and even the environment within your own vehicle all contribute to that risk. I still remember my high school Driver's Ed teacher, Mr. Gavrin, telling us over 30 years ago that "if you drive, you *will* eventually have an accident." He was right, of course, and I've unfortunately had several (although most of them were over twenty years ago, and not my fault), but driving is always risky—and something that requires care, attention, and vigilance every time you get behind the wheel.

Accidents will happen, of course—as Mr. Gavrin (and Elvis Costello) said. Some are more preventable, others perhaps not so much. But either way, accidents are costly, in terms of vehicular and property damage, physical injury, costs of treatment and related services, and time lost from work. Some statistics: In 2015, the last year for which data is available, there were 2.44 million people injured in vehicular accidents across the United States, with 35,000 deaths. According to the Department of Motor Vehicles, in New York State in 2015 there were 294,556 vehicle accidents (1,045 of them with fatalities), and 113,396 personal (bodily) injury claims. That's about 800 crashes every day. Insurance losses for that year in New York totaled $800,054,371. That's almost one billion dollars—in New York alone, in one year. The next year didn't fare any better, with 301,776 accidents (958 fatal) and 123,003 injury claims—an average of 826 accidents occurring daily. (Loss data for 2016 was not available.)

With so many accidents, insurance carriers are paying out billions of dollars a year, and the courts have full dockets of personal injury cases. But believe it or not, this system that we have today was instituted because the situation decades ago was believed to be even worse, and in many ways it was. Costs were out of control, and an accident case could take years to wend its way through the courts until a settlement was made and costs of treatment could be recovered. In an effort to control those costs and rein in delays, New York enacted a No-Fault system.

The No-Fault System: An Overview

New York State's automobile insurance system is the fourth largest in the country, with over 9 million vehicles insured and over 300 carriers vying to insure them; it's a 10 billion dollar business. The term "no-fault" refers to the reimbursement for any damages or injuries being made by each party's own insurer, regardless of which party is at fault for the accident. In other words, if John runs a stop sign and hits Bill, John's insurer will cover treatment of John's injuries and damage, and Bill's insurer will cover Bill's. Bill can sue John civilly for pain and suffering and lost work, and for injuries that meet the legal definition of a "serious" injury (see Chapter 3), but that is a proceeding that is separate from the "no-fault" system, and even though it is dealt with by the same insurers, it is handled by different departments and different adjusters. The latter deals with the at-fault party, while the former does not.

The no-fault system was instituted in 1974 to stem rapidly rising insurance costs and to streamline the process of compensation for treatment of auto accident injuries and damage, without requiring litigation. Prior to 1974, the courts were backlogged with the long, drawn-out process of handling claims, and reimbursement could often take years.

New York is one of twelve states, along with Puerto Rico, that have a "true" no-fault system, in that they impose certain thresholds and limits on claims and damages. Economic, or calculable, damages such as medical or funeral expenses and lost wages are capped at $50,000. If economic damages exceed $50,000, victims can go to court to recover them, along with other, non-economic damages such as emotional pain and suffering.

No-fault insurance travels along with the vehicle and covers all occupants of the particular vehicle. If a vehicle insured to John Doe in New York is involved in an accident in Pennsylvania, with 3 other passengers in the vehicle, John's policy will cover treatment of injuries to all four occupants, up to $50,000 for each occupant. No fault also covers injuries to pedestrians and bicyclists, who are entitled to "first party" benefits—meaning they have the same contractual right to coverage as the driver (who is the "first party"; the second and third parties being the insurance company and any other injured party, respectively). No-fault insurance does not cover taxis, motorcycles, or scooters, and does not cover injuries to a person resulting from them driving while intoxicated (DWI) or while engaged in other criminal activities. Additionally, no-fault coverage does not apply if the accident occurs during the course of the driver's employment, for example, a delivery vehicle or someone driving to multiple locations for work purposes. Such an accident would then be covered by Worker's Compensation.

Treatment Under No-Fault

Occupants of a covered vehicle who have sustained injuries while in an accident involving that vehicle may seek treatment for their injuries under the no-fault law. Section 5102(a)(1)(ii) of the New York Insurance Law provides for:

(1) All necessary expenses incurred for:
(i) medical, hospital (including services rendered in compliance with article forty-one of the public health law, whether or not such services are rendered directly by a hospital), surgical, nursing, dental, ambulance, x-ray, prescription drug and prosthetic services;

(ii) psychiatric, physical therapy (provided that treatment is rendered pursuant to a referral) and occupational therapy and rehabilitation;

(iii) any non-medical remedial care and treatment rendered in accordance with a religious method of healing recognized by the laws of this state; and

(iv) any other professional health services; all without limitation as to time, provided that within one year after the date of the accident causing the injury it is ascertainable that further expenses may be incurred as a result of the injury. For the purpose of determining basic economic loss, the expenses incurred under this paragraph shall be in accordance with the limitations of section five thousand one hundred eight of this article.

The law is fairly broadly written so that many different types of treatment are covered. Aside from medical care and physical therapy, other modalities such as, of course, chiropractic, as well as acupuncture, massage therapy, psychological care, audiology, and biofeedback are covered. It is fairly simple to begin the treatment process. A patient submits an Application for No Fault Benefits (Form NF-2), detailing the circumstances of the accident, to the insurer within 30 days. The patient and provider sign an Assignment of Benefits (Form NF-AOB), which transfers the patient's benefits and rights over to the provider—who can then directly submit claims for treatment to the insurer on the patient's behalf (via a standard HCFA form or an NF-3).

Relevant Regulations

If you're a practitioner treating patients under no-fault, you would do well to understand the basic framework of the system within which you are working. You don't have to become a legal expert in the system. That's what lawyers are for. But having a working knowledge of the regulations that are going to affect the patient's treatment and your, or your employer's, reimbursement will certainly be more than helpful; I can guarantee you that. Knowing the applicable regulations will let you know when and which forms, from both you and the patient, need to be submitted, deadlines for billing, and recourse in case of denial of payment.

The full text of the applicable laws and regulations can be found in the appendix of this book, as well as on the web via the links also supplied in the appendix.

Article 51—The No Fault Law

The "No-Fault" law, more technically known as Article 51 of the New York State Insurance Law, is officially titled the "Comprehensive Motor Vehicle Insurance Reparations Act." As was mentioned earlier, this law was promulgated in 1974 as a way of curbing out-of-control costs and delays in automobile accident insurance claims. In its nine sections, the Act sets forth the terms and definitions of coverage, what services and circumstances are and are not covered, sets limits on fees and charges, and provides for the exclusion of practitioners who have defrauded the system.

Regulation 83 & Regulation 68

The first version of the no-fault law had some problems, namely, practitioners treating injured patients/claimants were charging fees that were outrageously high. The entire point of the law was to curb costs and abuses of the system. Article 51 specifically provided for the establishment of a payment system, and Section 5108 of the law authorized the adoption of a fee schedule.

In December 1977, the Worker's Compensation Board established a fee schedule for medical, chiropractic, and other treatments and procedures for injured workers. Under Regulation 83 of the Insurance Law, this fee schedule was adopted into the no-fault law as well, as Regulation 68, although the other rules pertaining to the treatment of injured workers, such as requesting authorization for treatment, were not.

(A full history and text of Regulation 83 can be found at: http://www.dfs.ny.gov/insurance/r68/r83_intro.htm.)

The fee schedules are revised and updated periodically to reflect inflationary increases and new procedure codes (although if you ask most practitioners, not enough and not often enough).

Initially, chiropractic treatment under no-fault was not procedure-based but rather was reimbursed at a global rate. A chiropractic office visit in the New York metro area was reimbursed at a flat rate of $30.08 per visit until 1996, when it "jumped" to $33.70. Under this reimbursement structure, chiropractors were reimbursed the same fee whether they spent thirty minutes performing electrotherapy, myofascial work, ultrasound, and giving the patient exercises, or whether they gave the patient an adjustment that took two minutes. Only two main CPT codes were used: an initial office visit code—used once, typically 99203, and a follow-up visit code for all subsequent visits, typically 99213. This, of course, did not accurately reflect the actual procedure(s) done on a given visit.

In 2010, the fee schedule was completely overhauled and revised even further to reflect an RVU-based system. The RVU (Relative Value Unit) system is supposed to take into account the amount of work involved with a given procedure, as well the expenses of the provider and the average cost of practice in a given region. RVUs assign a value to each procedure code, which is then multiplied by a factor determined by profession and/or geographic region, to arrive at a dollar figure. This change allowed for more accurate representation of the actual procedures performed, as well as for a slight to modest increase in total visit fees, depending on the codes used. (A more detailed explanation of the RVU system can be found at:

http://medicaleconomics.modernmedicine.com/medical-economics/content/tags/calculating-relative-value-units/rvus-valuable-tool-aiding-practice-m?page=full.)

Regulation 68 also sets forth the timelines and deadlines within and by which the carrier must be notified of an intended claim, when an initial claim must be filed and when provider bills must be submitted, and which forms must be used. For example, claimants/patients are required to submit an Application for Benefits (form NF-2) within 30 days of the accident, and providers are required to send in their bills within 45 days. Regulation 68 has been amended a number of times between 2001 and 2017, to make changes to the application and billing timeframes and deadlines, clarify language, update forms, and debar certain providers from participation.

(A full history and the full text of Regulation 68 can be found at: http://www.dfs.ny.gov/insurance/r68/r68_new.htm.)

The No-Fault Industry and Flaws in the No-Fault System

Recall that basic no-fault coverage provides for injured parties to receive up to $50,000 in medical and other expenses, including 80 percent of income lost, up to $2000 a month. Also provided for are transportation costs to treatment and up to $25 a day in daily expense reimbursement. After the maximum $50,000 benefit has been exhausted, injured parties can take their claims to the courts to litigate further damages.

Now, $50,000 per person for treatment of injuries sounds like a good benefit—and it is. But unfortunately, many doctors, lawyers, and other practitioners saw this as something to be exploited.

Lawyers and doctors frequently have something of a symbiotic relationship within the no fault system. Doctors and clinics rely on lawyers to refer each other a steady stream of new accident patients. Lawyers rely on the providers to "build their cases"—to provide the documentation and the medical justification for lasting or "serious" injury and to meet or exceed the $50,000 benefit cap. Lawyers need this because, without evidence that their client sustained a legally serious enough injury that meets a certain economic threshold, there's nothing to litigate. That means no settlement for the client, and no reason for them to be involved; in other words, no money. Doctors and other providers will order and perform costly tests, therapies, and other procedures that will help do exactly that. Doctors (and chiropractors, and other providers), in turn, have their own economic interests to consider as well.

A practice prevalent in the industry is for attorneys' offices to partner with, or create, settlement funding firms that offer to advance funds to patients—sometimes many thousands of dollars—against their anticipated settlements. Patients may be happy to be getting so much money early on, but when the settlement comes, in addition to taking their rightful third, the attorneys or funding firms take back the loan amount *plus* the interest—sometimes leaving patients with relatively little.

As an example, one settlement funding firm advances $3,000.00 to a patient against their settlement. It charges a $285.00 "origination fee", and a $310.00 "underwriting fee". Interest is charged at the rate of 3.75%, compounded monthly. Just by walking out the door with the check, the patient owes $4483.61 (unless refunded within 5 days). After a year, the debt is $5591.86, and after 18 months it goes up to $6974.05. Given that many cases take at least that long to reach a settlement through the courts, funding companies are often making well over 100% profit. If a case settlement is only $20,000, it takes a significant chunk out of it—after repayment of the advance with interest and the attorney's cut, the patient is left with a little over $6000.00. While this is not illegal, and the terms are clearly spelled out in the funding contract, it is yet another way that money is generated by special interests in the industry.

No-fault is big business; as we have seen, the benefits available create a big pond from which many can "wet their beaks." Doctors, lawyers, therapists, drivers, technicians, suppliers of durable medical equipment (DME), imaging centers, managers, billers, and others all depend on the system for part, or often all, of their livelihoods. As a result, the costs involved in a given accident case can quickly soar. Everyone wants to get a piece of the pie. The no-fault system was designed to reduce and limit costs from auto accidents. The system is better than before 1974, to be sure. But opportunities for fraud, waste, and abuse are plenty.

2

CLINICS: THE LAY OF THE LAND

Thirty or forty years ago, most chiropractors practiced in solo offices or maybe shared their office with another practitioner or two. In the past twenty to twenty-five years, the landscape has changed. Many, if not most chiropractors working with personal-injury or no-fault patients (and even in more general practices) operate in a clinic-type setting. These clinics exist solely for the purpose of treating those injured in vehicular accidents. Some of them operate very appropriately and very well. Others do not; in fact, the situation can be quite the opposite.

The typical "no-fault clinic" setting is designed to maximize the services available and delivered to patients by combining multiple practitioners under one roof. Almost all no-fault clinics have a core of standard services: chiropractic, physical therapy, and acupuncture. Physical therapy is overseen by a medical physician, who patients see on their initial visit, and monthly thereafter for reevaluation and renewal of their physical therapy orders. These three services form the "bread and butter" of the therapeutic services provided.

Other specialty services provided include neurology, with specialized testing such as nerve conduction velocity (NCV) and electromyography (EMG); orthopedic and psychological services; computerized range-of-motion testing; and durable medical equipment and supplies such as cervical collars, braces, TENS electrical stimulators, plus pillows, cushions, and other sundry DME. Some clinics bring in biofeedback practitioners and chiropractors who perform manipulation under anesthesia (MUA).

Ideally, for a no-fault practice, making available all necessary services under one roof is a good model. It's easier to refer patients to specialists when necessary, it maintains continuity of care, and of course, it generates revenue for the clinic and its principals. Patients benefit when this model is set up and applied correctly. Is it always? No—and we will discuss that further later.

Chiropractors who practice no-fault are either self-employed in no-fault practice under their own sole proprietorship or Professional Corporation (P.C.) or work as an employee for a clinic or another chiropractor's P.C. Chiropractors can also be employed as a per diem or "coverage" doc, filling in for other chiropractors.

We'll talk about employee DCs a bit later, but one way self-employed chiropractors can set up in no-fault practice is to do so within their own existing general practice infrastructure. In this scenario, it's the chiropractor's practice and office, and the DC brings in a physical therapist, acupuncturist, and medical specialists to provide and supervise the necessary allied services. Typically, the DC sets up a separate P.C. that employs the MD and therapists, and the MD is named Medical Director of that P.C. Alternatively, an MD with his own P.C. rents space within the DC's office. The DC provides the chiropractic care, and chiropractic and non-chiropractic services are billed separately under their respective PCs.

Under this kind of arrangement, the DC maintains more control over the patient sourcing or procurement, as well as personnel, being the director of the business. However, this kind of practice may also be costlier and require more effort for the DC to set up legally.

The other common type of scenario is essentially the reverse of the first one; a DC joins a clinic that already has an existing infrastructure. Here, the clinic is already set up. An MD with his own P.C. is medical director of the clinic, which may have managers that oversee the billing and other non-medical operations. The physical therapist is employed by the MD, and other providers such as the acupuncturist and chiropractor rent space under their respective P.C.s.

It should be noted that in both scenarios, any leasing or rental of space in another's facility must be at fair market value. For example, a clinic's management can't ask for 50% of a DC's billings under the guise of renting him a $1200 office for $5000. That's thinly disguised fee-splitting, it won't stand up to scrutiny, and it can land both parties in legal trouble.

Chiropractic and medical services should be billed separately as described above because they are different licenses, and neither can do what the other can. In other words, an MD can employ another medical physician, because they both have the same license. An MD can employ a physical therapist because the MD orders and supervises the physical therapy. But an MD cannot oversee chiropractic care because an MD is not a chiropractor. Conversely, a DC cannot practice medicine. So, under state law, an MD cannot employ a chiropractor. There may be some allowance for a medical corporation (PC) to employ a DC, with certain caveats. Anyone considering entering either kind of arrangement should consult an attorney with experience in these areas.

Positives and Negatives

Throughout almost 25 years of practice, I have worked in different capacities in my career; I have been employed as an associate in a number of general as well as no-fault clinics; I have worked for many years as a cover (or "temp") doctor, where I would fill in for a day or two, or a week, in a clinic where the regular doctor was out, or where the clinic was between permanent doctors; and I have owned a private practice, sharing space with a medical physician in his large clinic and physical therapy center where there were a significant number of no fault patients. So, with apologies to Sergio Leone, while I have seen the good results of no-fault practice, I have also seen its "bad and ugly" attributes; no-fault practice has many positive aspects, but also has negatives.

The Good

From a chiropractic perspective, no-fault injury practice opens up access to an entire demographic of patients who have never had chiropractic care and probably otherwise never would. Many patients in no-fault clinics are poor, un- or under-employed, and are not native English speakers. Some have no other health insurance coverage or are covered by Medicaid, which does not provide a chiropractic benefit. Many patients in no-fault clinics do not have a regular physician or do not see one regularly. So, chiropractors are in a unique position to deliver care to a niche of the population that is generally underserved in health care in general, and not served with chiropractic at all. As first-access providers, a DC may be the first such provider that an accident patient will see upon entering the clinic. The patient may have undiagnosed hypertension, diabetes, or other insidious and chronic ailments that a chiropractor would be able to, with proper interviewing and examination, detect and refer to the appropriate provider. This is unquestionably a good thing, since patients can get care they otherwise would not have.

The clinic model of practice, combining chiropractic, medical, and other allied services is, of course, a good idea. A patient who comes to the clinic after an auto accident complaining of pain in the neck, back, shoulder, and knee can have his or her complaints evaluated and followed by different specialists, and receive therapy, imaging, and even surgery, without having to be "referred out." There is continuity of the patient's care across different specialties. There is a unified medical and care record, or at least easy access to different practitioners' records.

As an example of what a good no-fault clinic should be, for several years I worked in a clinic that was 99% no-fault (the other 1% being Worker's Compensation, which I was not involved with). I found this office after too many years working in offices like the other ones you will see described later.

The physical facility was well-kept. It wasn't beautiful—no fancy fixtures, wall moldings, or artwork—but it was built out well, clean as a whistle, and well maintained. The equipment was top-notch—in fact, they purchased a brand-new Leander motorized flexion traction table, with full drops and adjustability. While patient volume was moderate and could be high at times, the flow of patients was orderly and efficient. There was enough staff, and good equipment in the physical therapy area as well. Patients completed regular monthly Oswestry and other questionnaires. Patient visit frequency was monitored and tailored to improvement, and there was frequent communication between and among the different providers.

When implemented properly, the clinic model is a good way to ensure that patients who have injuries resulting from vehicular accidents receive quality treatment that is tailored to their type of injury, by professionals who are experienced, in an appropriate setting, that is organized and compliant with legal, ethical, and professional standards and guidelines. But like any otherwise good idea, it can also be implemented poorly and improperly—and sometimes fraudulently, as we'll see a bit later.

The Bad

We'll use "bad" to refer to things like poor business and recordkeeping habits, sloppy clinical practices, run-down facilities and poor equipment, and other similar lapses or distasteful situations, while "ugly" we'll reserve for more nefarious issues, like fraud. The "bad" and "ugly" sides of no-fault exist where the only goal is to make money. When you take pride in your office, in your profession, and in the services you provide—and when you genuinely care for the people you see—the issues described below won't really apply.

First, let's talk about the "bad" rather than the "ugly" category; again, "bad" being a relative term and "ugly" being reserved for issues more of a fraudulent nature. Here are some general descriptions of typical "bad" clinics, based on many of my part-time and per-diem experiences. And again, let's be clear that while highly prevalent in the industry, not every clinic falls into this category, although some may fall into both.

Location, Location, Location

Most no-fault clinics in this category are in poorer, more urban areas—some very urban, and by that I mean places where you might not want to walk alone at night, like south Jamaica, parts of the Bronx, and East New York. It's not always easy to park there, and if there's alternate-side parking, you could spend 30 minutes circling to find an open legal spot.

There are likely several reasons for this. First, commercial space there is less costly. Also, much of the clinic's patient base comes from the surrounding geographic area, and convenience makes it easier for patients to make regular visits.

A Typical Clinic

Many offices themselves are frequently in less than pristine condition. Often the clinic is a storefront, with a waiting area in front and a large therapy "gym" and several treatment rooms in the back. In better clinics of this type, the rooms are fully divided, with a door that closes (although the room can be pretty small; I can recall rooms where there wasn't enough space for me to walk around the table). In some of the clinics I've worked in, the room's walls didn't fully reach the ceiling, and in a few that I can recall, the chiropractic treatment area was just a table in a corner of the therapy area, with a curtain or a portable screen/divider for privacy. There might be a poster or two on the walls—usually the "whiplash" and "spine disorders" ones that we're all familiar with.

The therapy area usually has at least four therapy tables surrounded by hospital-style curtains, each with electrical stim machines. There are a couple of desks or a large desk area where the PT and acupuncturist will sit. There will also likely be an array of physical therapy equipment, like a recumbent bike or an ergometer, a treadmill, weights, and maybe a shoulder wheel. But in my experience, in most clinics, these things are rarely, if ever, used. (I don't think I can ever recall seeing a patient on a treadmill.)

In the chiropractor's room, the adjustment table is almost always an old bench table, frequently with torn vinyl upholstery and a broken paper holder. In many offices, there isn't even any chiropractic face paper—just a loose roll of long therapy table paper.

The desk is usually small enough to be able to fit in an already small room along with a treatment table, and sometimes a two- or four- drawer vertical filing cabinet (more on records in Chapter 14).

Below are examples of some of the no-fault clinics I have encountered. I highly doubt any of them are still in operation at this time.

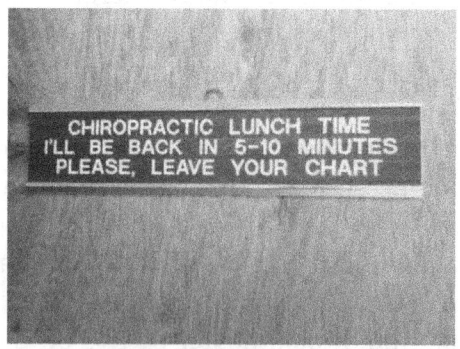

This was the sign on the door to the chiropractic treatment room in one clinic where I did a coverage job. I thought it was hilarious—you can almost hear the Russian accent as you read it. Apparently, there were so many patients in this clinic daily, the regular doctor felt he couldn't go to lunch for 5 minutes without missing someone.

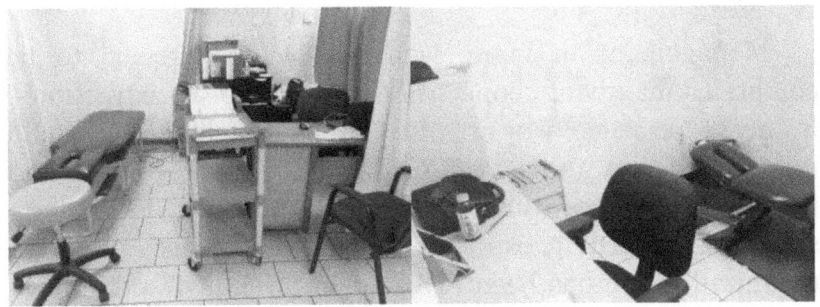

Actual chiropractic treatment areas in typical clinics I covered. Note that the one on the left is not an actual room, but just a corner of the clinic with curtains. (See the anecdote on "unperformed services" in Chapter 3 for more about that clinic.) The clinic on the right was located in a storefront in Brooklyn, with dirty walls that did not reach the ceiling, and dead roaches on the floor.

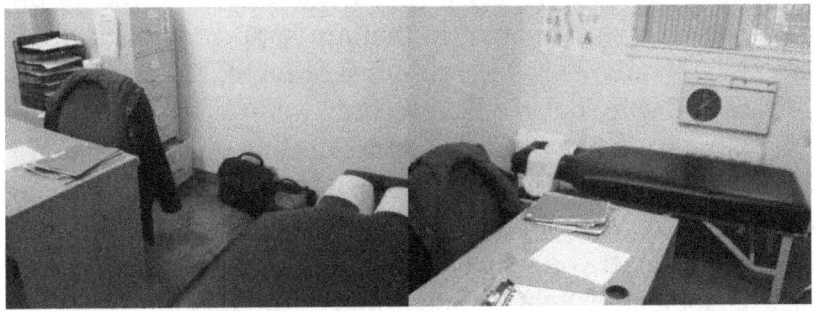

This was a clinic I did a 2 or 3-day coverage job for sometime in the mid 2000s, where I saw an average of about 90 patients per day. The clinic took up the entire basement area of an apartment building in East New York, Brooklyn; there were low ceilings and exposed pipes. The chiropractic treatment area was just a space between two short hallways, with no doors or curtains to close. I was offered more work there but declined.

Management

Management in many New York clinics seems to be comprised mainly of people of Eastern European extraction—in my experience working in dozens of clinics, I would estimate that in about 90% of them, the clinic owners and managers were of that background. I found this to be somewhat unsettling, especially since it is known that Russian organized crime has been involved in no-fault fraud, and in many recent media cases of no-fault fraud, the majority of the perpetrators were Eastern European, as we shall see later.

In many clinics, there are cameras in the reception and in the public areas as well as outside, and there is often one room—usually a back office—that is kept locked. Sometimes it has an electronic keypad lock, and a camera as well. This is the business office, where the clinic owners and principals come and go. I've never gone in there, nor have I ever really wanted to. But the secrecy begs the question as to the nature of the meetings and activities that are happening back there. It's understandable to lock an office at night, to keep records private and safe, but medical records weren't kept there, and after all, it's not like these clinics are dealing in cash. On many occasions, I have observed Russian-speaking men driving expensive Mercedeses and BMWs coming and going from these rooms, dressed in designer jeans, shoes, and leather jackets, looking like they came from Central Casting.

Sometime early in my career, I was called by a doctor I had worked for in the past to cover a clinic in Brooklyn. The office was in a fairly decent neighborhood, near where I'd spent part of my childhood. I'd been here before. What I mean is, I actually had been here before, in this very office; I'd worked a per diem job here about 5 years prior, when it had been under different management. Not much else had changed, though, from the looks of things.

As is typically the case in clinics of this type, the place was pretty rundown. My treatment "room" was a cramped and windowless 6 ½ X 12 space with a treatment table, an office chair and small desk, and a file cabinet. The table looked to be the same one that had been there about 5 years ago, only with more duct tape patching the cracks in the vinyl.

The office was already thronged with patients when I arrived at 9:30. The morning crowd was all comprised of elderly Russians, bused in by the management; think Moscow In Bensonhurst. Immediately, I plunged in, seeing several new patients. Not speaking any Russian, I relied on gesticulation, saying things louder, and whatever rudimentary English the patient knew ("Pain? Where is pain? Here? Here?"); I mostly got by, except in one case where I had to call in one of the staff to translate (a Russian woman with coiffed hair and 5-inch spiked heels that were, literally, spikes; a 5-inch metal rod with a ball on the end). I prayed I hadn't missed anything important. I took solace in the fact that I was only subbing- and that the regular doc would reexamine them when he returned, and that whatever treatment I'd be doing would be very low-force anyway. With one man, I couldn't complete his intake because there was no one to translate.

I couldn't even find a reflex hammer.

The place was noisy and crowded. Forget HIPAA. Those waiting next in line stood and gawked at their comrades under my earnest ministrations. One man insisted on removing his shoes and socks and having me click my adjusting instrument on his feet. (And managed to do it without a word of English, too.)

It was easier to just do it and click a few random spots than to argue.

After about 90 minutes and about a third as many difficult-to-pronounce surnames, things settled down to a more manageable steady trickle. Since there was no internet connection (I really didn't expect one, though sometimes you get lucky), I didn't have much else to do but read yesterday's paper and practice my hook shot from my desk with the used face paper.

I stepped out to get a breath of air and some natural light and observed a knot of shaven-headed and black-leathered men clustered around a gleaming black BMW SUV. Amid a cloud of cigarette smoke, they spoke in Russian and clapped one another on the shoulders in a way not just a little reminiscent of The Sopranos. I gazed around blithely, munching an apple. It wasn't hard to do the math.

One of the patients I saw that afternoon entered the room dressed in green scrubs. I joked that now I didn't feel like the only one wearing pajamas. I asked her where she worked.

"Mount Sinai", she said, referring to the hospital.

"What do you do there?" I countered.

"I'm a fourth-year medical student."

My eyebrows went up. "This may sound like a dumb question," I asked, "but.... what are you doing here?"

She smiled and shrugged. "Car accident, like everyone else."

I lowered my voice a notch. "Well, obviously," I replied. "But I mean- what are you doing..." I gestured around the cramped room, "here?"

"Oh, well, one of my family members is involved with running this place, you know, so... like they say- loyalties run deep."

"I see," I said, noticing the surname on her chart. "But you understand why I asked."

"Of course," she replied. "And you understand my answer."

I'm not sure what that says about her. Or medicine. But she said that she was going to do her residency in reconstructive surgery, and she actually thought highly of chiropractors and felt benefit from the treatment. I saw 64 patients that day.

Very often, chiropractors get into an arrangement with a clinic's management that typically goes something like this: the clinic owners/managers offer a DC space in the clinic, along with access to all the clinic's patients. In other words, the DC will have a room in the clinic and all patients coming into the clinic after a car accident will see the DC for treatment, along with the rest of the providers in the office.

Ideally, and legally, this should only be a straightforward rental arrangement, with the DC paying a market rate for his room and use of common areas, and patients given the choice of seeing the DC. However, all the patients are steered to the

DC, and in exchange, management wants a percentage of the DC's billing receivables; this is, of course, illegal under various state and Federal laws against fee-splitting, and may also be considered as the DC being a "straw owner" (more on that later). So, to disguise this practice, often the clinic management will make the DC's tenancy contingent on also handling the DC's billing for him/her, and taking a large cut of the chiropractor's receivables, accounting it as payment for "billing" and/or "marketing" services.

Patients

The patients in these types of clinics are usually representative of the demographic and culture of the surrounding areas and are usually working-class, or sometimes unemployed. Generally, they are pleasant to deal with, though in my experience patients from some cultures are more compliant and respectful than others. There can be patients that seem disinterested in their care, and those that actually seem somewhat sullen, but most are agreeable enough.

No-fault clinics don't schedule appointments. Unless a patient needs to see a specialist that is only there on a particular day, patients are simply told to come for treatment 3-4 days per week anytime during clinic hours (typically between 10AM-noon and 8PM). This can result in some busy periods if many patients decide to come around the same time. The hours after 5PM are typically always busy, when the patients who are working will come in.

Patient volume in most no-fault clinics is typically high—although some offices see around 30 patients per day, there are offices that see twice, or even three times, that number. Higher volume clinics are obviously less comfortable to work in. Higher volume clinics (above 60 chiropractic patient visits per day) are also more likely to be involved with suspicious activity, and I would recommend not working in those facilities. We will discuss patient volume further in Chapter 16.

Employers

When chiropractors work for other chiropractors, as I have for many years, often it is the employer DCs themselves that are "bad." Very often these employer DCs are nothing more than absentee bosses who rent space in a clinic (as I described above)—or two or three—and then plug associate doctors into them to see the patients (read: generate billing). Sometimes these employer DCs seem to care very little about how the patients are treated. They just need a warm body with a valid license to do something chiropractic to the patient and to make sure there is a record of it with the appropriate "i"s dotted and "t"s crossed so as not to delay reimbursement. They also don't much care how the employee doctor is treated; hours can be long (usually around ten-hour days), and patient volume can be quite high. It is not unusual for a DC in a no-fault clinic to see upward of 40 or 50 patients in one day. For this reason, there seems to be a very high rate of employee DC turnover in no-fault clinics—no one seems to want to do it for very long. There are always job ads posted for chiropractors on the various chiropractic internet job boards, and often the same employers are posting every few months. It's good for getting work (including coverage work), but it's a sad commentary on chiropractic working conditions and how employers treat employee doctors.

Some less scrupulous employer chiropractors also seem to have trouble paying employee doctors on time. I and other colleagues have had checks bounce or be late, and there were coverage jobs where I had to repeatedly call the employer doc for weeks and ask when payment would be made. Fortunately, such employers are not the norm. However, I would recommend that for any per diem coverage job, whether it's for a single day or two weeks, ask for payment up front, even a post-dated check. If you're to be paid on a W-2, it probably won't be possible to be paid up front, but you can ask for direct deposit into your bank account.

If you're a chiropractor who employs other chiropractors to work in your clinic, pay them fairly and on time. Don't ask them to do something you yourself wouldn't do, or even more importantly, shouldn't do. Following an employer's instructions can get someone in very big legal trouble and is not a defense; we will examine that later on.

Should you work for these clinics?

The best way to enter into no-fault practice as a principal in this type of clinic setting would be to do it the first way that was mentioned earlier—in your own facility, bringing in the other providers and maintaining greater business and clinical control. But either way, chiropractors who want to enter into no-fault practice for themselves, and want to practice in a space-sharing type of clinic setting, should be extremely careful about it. Know who you are getting involved with, get all the terms on paper beforehand, and have everything reviewed by an attorney with experience in healthcare law and healthcare business organization. If you encounter resistance from the clinic owners and managers regarding anything that should be handled in a straightforward manner, that should be enough indication to avoid involvement and seek an arrangement elsewhere.

It should obviously go without saying that you must never, ever enter into an illegal business arrangement with another party. If you are a DC considering a space-rental agreement with a clinic, keep everything above board. You should only agree to pay—and actually pay—a fair market rate for the space you use, that is in line with similar rates based on square footage in your area. No fee-splitting, no payments based on patient volume or patients referred, and if the clinic management does your billing, it should be based on prevailing rates in the industry, such as an hourly or per-claim rate, or even a flat monthly rate that does not vary.

If you are a DC who is not in a position to open your own practice, or if you are building your practice but need to supplement your income, you will need to work for another established chiropractor to make ends meet. Because no-fault clinics are so prevalent in the metropolitan area (remember what I said earlier about half the profession disappearing overnight?), chances are pretty good that you will be working in a no-fault clinic—at least at some point.

If you are an employee DC, either as a full or part-time associate or as a covering doctor, you obviously have no control over the business arrangements of your employer. However, it is important to be aware of the prevalent bad practices and to watch out for them, because they will frequently come up.

The Ugly

Here we come to the darker side of no-fault practice: fraud. Of course, no-fault practice can be, and often is, done appropriately and legally. But there is a deep vein of fraud that runs throughout the industry, and as the statistics show, it is only getting worse.

Hopefully, no one goes through the long and difficult journey of obtaining a professional degree with the intent of using it to commit fraud; we all (again, hopefully!) start out with noble intentions. We enter helping professions to help people. So how is it that too many chiropractors—and medical doctors and others—end up becoming involved in fraud?

I'm not a sociologist, but I have several theories. There are all kinds of people in society; some people are natural "wheeler-dealers"; they're always looking to game the system, and see the law as something to be followed only if it doesn't prevent them from getting what they want. There are people like this who go to chiropractic school too. They don't really love chiropractic . . . if they did, they wouldn't abuse it for personal gain. To them, it's just an avenue toward benefitting themselves, a means to an end.

Then there are the doctors who may start out with noble intentions, but find it difficult to make ends meet "playing by the book." So they make a deal with the devil, and get involved with crooked or questionable people and situations. And they'll tell themselves they're just doing what everyone else does, what they have to do, because otherwise you can't make any money in this business. They tell themselves they're really only *bending* the law—maybe—not breaking it, right?

And finally, there are those doctors who get caught up in unethical behavior without the predetermination to do so. They might be an employee of another doctor or clinic involved with unethical and/or illegal practices, and they figure they aren't responsible. Maybe they look the other way and rationalize that whatever it is that might be a problem isn't really a problem, or that it's only an isolated instance instead of a pattern. This is really the most dangerous and insidious type of fraud situation, because the person involved doesn't even think he or she is.

As a Doctor of Chiropractic, it is imperative to uphold the highest ethical and professional standards of care. It can be too easy to get involved with something illegal that may seem to be just a simple and lucrative practice and business opportunity that so many other chiropractors are also doing, or to take a position as an employee doctor in a clinic, and look the other way and not ask too many questions when ethical issues arise (and they will). If you're a person who is intent on bending or breaking the law, you may be beyond the kind of help this book can offer. But if you're honest, and want to practice honorably and ethically, a major part of avoiding fraudulent practices and situations is knowing what they are and what to look for, and that is what the following section of this book will help you do.

NO-FAULT WITH NO FEAR

II

THE FRAUD FACTOR

"Fraud is the daughter of greed."
—Jonathan Gash, *The Great California Game*

"The path of least resistance leads to crooked rivers and crooked men."
—Henry David Thoreau

"The man who is admired for the ingenuity of his larceny is almost always rediscovering some earlier form of fraud. The basic forms are all known, have all been practiced. The manners of capitalism improve. The morals may not."
—John Kenneth Galbraith

NO-FAULT WITH NO FEAR

3

FRAUD AND ITS FORMS

As long as there have been primitive societies, there has been fraud. Since the first cavemen began trading sticks for animal hides, people have been trying to cheat and steal from one another. The Bible enjoins against it, in the Ten Commandments, no less.

The earliest recorded case of insurance fraud is said to have occurred in the third century B.C. in ancient Greece (the ancient Greeks invented insurance—and then promptly invented insurance fraud), and involved a type of maritime insurance known as "bottomry." Bottomry was a form of insurance where the master of a sailing or cargo ship would borrow money against it, or "upon its bottom." If the ship was lost at sea (as would sometimes happen), the lender would lose the loan. If the ship made it to port, the borrower would repay the loan with interest, at a much higher than normal rate known as "maritime interest," because of the higher risk to the lender. If the loan was not repaid, the ship and its cargo, or their value, would be forfeited as collateral. This type of early insurance likely arose out of ship captains' need to pay for repairs to their vessels in foreign ports, and in order to preserve cash flow would use these loans to maintain their vessels, sell their cargo at a profit, and then repay the loan.

A sea merchant named Hegestratos took out a bottomry loan against his ship, with a cargo of corn, to sail from Syracuse (now Sicily) to Athens. However, Hegestratos never really planned to reach Athens; he, along with his partner Xenothermios, planned to sink their cargo-less ship, escape back to shore on a raft, and keep the loan against their (overvalued) vessel and its non-existent cargo. Their plan was—well, sunk—when the crew discovered Heggy down in the empty hold trying to drill a hole through the hull. Naturally, they were quite upset that he was willing to drown them to make a few coins, and to escape them, Heggy jumped overboard and was drowned.

It was actually quite common for merchant mariners to take out bottomry loans and then claim their ships were sunk, all the while hiding them in a foreign port. In fact, such schemes were probably contrived as soon as bottomry loans came into being. This practice became known as "ship scuttling" and continued well into the 19th and 20th centuries. What makes this case noteworthy for its time is that Hegestratos was caught in the act. Sadly, fraudulent conduct has not changed in the millennia since Hegestratos. As with bottomry, fraud has been a problem in the no-fault industry practically since no-fault insurance was instituted.

No-Fault Fraud

Fraud is a very real, very pervasive, and very resistant problem in no-fault. It exists in different forms, and often several different parties are involved. It's always been around, although it has been getting worse; in the last 5 years, cases of no-fault fraud have increased over 800 percent. Cases of no-fault fraud in New York increased from 400 in 1991 to almost 10,000 cases by 1998, and between 1994 and 1997, arrests for insurance fraud increased one and a half times.[1] No-fault fraud can be thought of in terms of both "soft" fraud, like obtaining patients through questionable sources, overstatement of injuries, over-treatment, and over-testing; and "hard" fraud, such as staging accidents, unnecessary treatment, and false billing (i.e. no-show visits and services not performed).

Fraud increases the costs of insurance to policyholders. It is estimated that the "cost of fraud" per family is somewhere between $200 and $700. Additionally, the costs of treatment and the average bodily injury claim is higher in New York than in any other state.

Part of the problem is that the system is very open to exploitation; the rules in the no-fault laws, specifically the Comprehensive Motor Vehicle Insurance Reparations Act, or VRA, state that an insurer has thirty days from receipt of a claim to pay or deny the claim—known as the "thirty-day rule." The purpose of the rule was to quickly and expediently resolve injury claims, so that accident victims could be quickly reimbursed for medical and other expenses. The rules allow a claimant to assign his or her policy benefits to medical providers, so that the providers are reimbursed directly. Many clinics will bombard insurers with multiple claims for medical and other examinations, various treatment modalities, tests, transportation, etc., and the insurer will not have time to conduct a thorough investigation into the claims before the allowed thirty days have elapsed. (The thirty days can be

---

[1] Papa, L. and Basile, A.. (2016). No Fault Insurance Fraud: An Overview. Touro Law Review, 17(3), p.2.

delayed while the carrier requests missing information, but smart clinics will send in all necessary information to begin the claims process right away.)

Runners

Virtually all dedicated no-fault clinics build their patient base through the use of "runners" (also called "drivers," or "cappers"). Runners are people who monitor police radio frequencies for reports of vehicle collisions, then appear on the scene and helpfully approach the victims to offer their assistance and services. (I'm not sure how they decide to which party to offer their assistance, but I'm guessing there is some assessment made as to which party is more likely at fault, and the runners approach the other.) Another tactic of runners is to obtain the contact information of parties involved in an accident from the police accident reports, which legally are public information, and call the victims claiming to work with "the insurance," or "a clinic that deals with your insurance" (of course it does), or other vague representations. They assure the involved party that they will take care of everything—take them to a clinic to treat their injuries, take care of their vehicle, help them with their insurance claims, "hook them up" with a lawyer—and that they might well have a case against the other party which could result in a nice payday for them. Not surprisingly, many accident victims accept this arrangement. It's also not surprising that in many clinics, a good number of the patients are low-income, poorly or uneducated, or unemployed (although some are working-class and employed). Runners are typically paid somewhere in the neighborhood of $1000–$1500 per patient referred (usually after the patient has visited the clinic a certain number of times, and/or had certain costly tests), and are paid under the table. Probably the best indicator that a clinic is using runners is when a patient visits the clinic on the same day the accident occurred—sometimes, within hours.

So, you may ask, what's the problem with runners? Accidents are often terribly stressful ordeals. Aren't there are some people who might appreciate a helpful guide to get them treatment and steer them through the no-fault system after an accident disrupts their lives?

Well, yes. But the problem is that runners are financially incentivized. Again, runners typically get paid once the patient has visited a clinic a certain number of times, ensuring that the clinic doesn't lose money on the patient. This can result in runners "suggesting" to potential patients that a certain length of treatment or number of visits is necessary, and perhaps coaching them on how to describe their injuries. Some patients may embellish or exaggerate their symptoms. (If you are observant, you may notice patients whose range of motion upon examination seems just a bit more limited than before or after the exam, or a numerical pain rating given that is inconsistent with their behavior—i.e., the patient claims his pain is a 9/10—10 being described as excruciating, like childbirth or a kidney stone—while sitting calmly and in no apparent distress.)

Believe it or not, using runners is not strictly illegal; there is nothing in the New York statutes that explicitly prohibits this. Providers paying for patient referrals is, of course, illegal, especially with regard to Medicare and other commercial forms of health care, and it is also illegal in New York for lawyers to pay for referrals from non-lawyers. But while it may well be questionable ethically, since the providers themselves are not directly compensating anyone for the referral, it can get a little nebulously gray.

There have been recent efforts to make using runners to acquire accident patients illegal. In 2013, a bill (S424) was introduced to the Senate in the New York State Legislature to criminalize acting as a runner or soliciting or employing a runner to procure patients or clients. The bill would make violations of the anti-runner law a class D felony. As of this writing, the bill has passed the Senate and has been delivered to the Assembly. If it passes the Assembly as well, it will be delivered to the Governor to be either signed into law or vetoed. I'm not so sure that passing this bill into law is a "slam dunk"; New York has a very powerful lawyer's lobby, and as you might imagine, personal injury lawyers stand to lose quite a bit if this bill were to pass. (Chiropractors would also stand to lose quite a bit as well—remember what I said earlier about half the profession disappearing overnight? Time will tell, of course.)

Overtreatment and Overutilization

This is another form of "soft" fraud that occurs very frequently in no-fault practice. Patients are often seen (usually three times per week on average) until their treatment is terminated by the IME (independent medical examination), and sometimes beyond—even when such frequency may not be supported by their subjective complaints and objective findings. The patient is re-evaluated monthly by the medical physician to update their physical therapy orders, and told to continue. Most clinics provide transportation services, so patients are driven to and from the office, which helps to ensure that most patients follow the schedule. Many patients are also over diagnosed on their initial visit, and given diagnosis codes for radiculopathy when they only have local pain and no radicular signs or symptoms. Patients are often also given multiple diagnostic tests for every area of even the slightest complaint— MRIs, nerve conduction tests and EMGs, computerized range-of-motion tests, etc. This practice of over diagnosis, over testing, and overtreatment is known in the insurance industry as "buildup."

Certainly, many patients have complaints and findings that justify diagnostic tests and a maintained visit frequency; perhaps even most do. But some do not, and continuing to rubber-stamp the same orders for diagnostic tests for every patient, and to treat them without at least a trial of reduced frequency contributes to inflated and unnecessary costs.

Example: A 26-year-old man presents 3 days after a rear and left-sided vehicle collision. He had no loss of consciousness and did not go to the hospital. He complains of mild to moderate neck pain to his upper shoulders, and mild low back pain at the waist that does not radiate. The pain is mild but becomes moderate after sitting longer than 30 minutes. He denies any paresthesias in any extremities. He is employed as a manager and did not miss any work. On exam, he has 80% of normal range of motion in all planes with mild end range pain. His cervical and lumbosacral muscles are mildly tender and hypertonic. He has no sensory, motor, or reflex deficit, and straight leg raise causes mild lower back pain only at 70 degrees. He has mild local neck pain upon shoulder depression and Soto-Hall maneuvers. Chiropractic subluxations are palpated in the cervical and lumbar spine.

Pretty straightforward findings, no? Mild local symptoms only, and no indication whatsoever of radiculopathy. Yet a patient like this may typically be ordered physical therapy 3–4 times per week—which goes on for three or four months—and immediately be given orders for cervical and lumbar MRIs. MRIs are typically reviewed by the insurer (which includes requesting notes and examination findings), to determine if sufficient time was allowed for healing to take place and if the MRI was still necessary (typically 4–6 weeks from the date of accident). Even if his symptoms are improving by the time the imaging is scheduled, the MRIs are usually done anyway. MRI findings, even of questionable significance like bulges or small herniations that do not correlate to complaints, are then used to justify further treatment and testing, such as costly and painful EMGs.

Of course, there are patients who are seriously injured and whose continued symptomatology and/or objective findings warrant ongoing treatment and diagnostic testing. Also, this kind of overutilization can be difficult to put a finger on. As doctors of chiropractic, we are trained early to view the spine as requiring ongoing maintenance, and chiropractic adjustments as something that does not necessarily end; it becomes very easy to fall into a pattern of continuing to adjust a patient two or three times per week indefinitely, when they may need it less often. It may not seem like a big difference, but multiplied across the entire industry it becomes a significant cost factor. Ideally, chiropractors should be tailoring their treatment, visit frequency, and diagnostic tests to the individual patient, and be using objective methods to that end, such as regular outcomes assessment questionnaires (i.e., Oswestry, etc.) and detailed re-examinations.

One problem is that attorneys want data that supports their case; remember that the attorney needs to establish a "serious injury" in order to bring a suit for pain and suffering in a New York court.

"Serious injury" is defined under Article 51 (NYCRR § 5102(d)) as:

> "Serious injury" means a personal injury which results in (1) death, (2) dismemberment,(3) significant disfigurement, (4) fracture, (5) loss of a fetus, (6) permanent and total loss of use of a body organ, member, function, or system, (7) permanent consequential limitation of use of a body organ or member, (8) significant limitation of use of a body function or system, and (9) a medically determined injury or impairment of a non-permanent nature which prevents the injured person from performing substantially all of the material acts which constitute such person's usual and customary daily activities for not less than 90 days during the 180 days immediately following the occurrence of the injury or impairment.

Most of these criteria (1–6) are self-explanatory. The issues arise when establishing criteria 7–9, which require objective evidence beyond complaints of pain alone. Even treatment notes recording the presence of spasm may not be sufficient, but if spasm can be established by an objective test, then that could support "serious injury." Even a herniated disc by itself does not establish "serious injury"—unless it can be shown objectively that the herniation is causing a physical limitation, and then the doctor must state to what degree that limitation exists. So, every patient is given a gamut of tests (MRIs; EMGs; computerized range of motion tests; and functional capacity evaluations, or FCEs) in what seems to be less of an effort to direct patient care than to generate data that attorneys need to allow them to bring a case to court. Ironically, the no-fault laws, such as the one above, were supposed to *reduce* litigation and congestion in the courts by weeding out non-serious injuries. Unfortunately, it's not very difficult to see that instead of the clinical interests of the patient, what drives clinical decisions in many no-fault clinics is instead the financial interests of multiple parties—clinic managers, attorneys, runners, the patients themselves, and even clinical professionals. It is that symbiosis of financial gain among everyone involved that leads to the creation of the kind of clinic where this occurs—the "mill."

No-Fault "Mills"

Over the last twenty-five years or so, there has been a proliferation of clinics in the New York metropolitan area referred to by many as "mills"—as in, the clinic is a "mill" that patients are fed into and that churns out claims. Mills typically see very high volumes of patients and generate tens of thousands of dollars in bills per patient, often for services that are unnecessary and in some cases, not even rendered. Recent cases in the media of mass arrests for no-fault fraud have involved such mills, which are frequently connected to Russian organized crime. In a mill, the "MO." generally follows the formula described earlier—runners working for mill owners, and sometimes attorneys, recruit accident claimants/patients to visit the mill; runners are paid up to $1500 for each patient recruited. Attorneys associated with the mill may be directly involved with its operations, or may be looking the other way at injuries they know are likely magnified and fabricated. Attorneys may make payments for referrals under the guise of paying for "medical records." Medical providers may simply be relying on patients' descriptions of their symptoms of pain and basic exam findings to justify more extensive testing and treatment, or they may be more unscrupulously rubber-stamping tests and treatments on all patients. Some doctors (and chiropractors) are more involved in the mill operations, and some accept a regular payment from mill owners to "use" their medical license numbers to bill for services, without or hardly ever actually seeing patients. Patients themselves may not be aware that their claims are being used as cash cows for the mill, or they may be in on the scam, sometimes being paid several hundred dollars to visit the mill a set number of times.

In the most egregious cases, mill owners will actually stage, or cause the accidents they are billing for. There are a variety of ways this is done. One method is for a runner to recruit several people, who may not even know each other. These recruits, usually at least three, get into an old clunker car and drive to a predetermined location where they purposely cause a minor crash with an unsuspecting motorist (a favorite technique is the "swoop and squat," where the runner vehicle cuts in front of the target vehicle and suddenly brakes, causing the target vehicle to hit it from behind), or they feign a collision with another recruit involved in the scheme. Another way is to call a car service and have another conspirator cause an accident with it. There are many variations on these techniques.

The National Insurance Crime Bureau (NICB) has published a list of possible indicators of the kind of fraudulent claims and treatments that may be produced by a mill:[2]

1. Three or more occupants in the claimant's vehicle, all of whom report similar injuries.

2. All injuries are subjectively diagnosed, such as headaches, muscle spasms, traumas, and inability to sleep.

3. Minor accident produces major medical costs, lost wages and unusually expensive demands for pain and suffering.

4. All of the claimants submit medical bills from the same doctor or medical facility.

5. Medical bills submitted are photocopies of the originals.

6. Summary medical bills are submitted without dates and descriptions of office visits and treatments, or treatment extends for a lengthy period without any interim bills.

7. Vehicle driven by claimant is an old clunker with minimal coverage.

8. Insured, even though legally liable for the accident, is adamant that claimants were responsible for the accident, indicating that the insured may have been targeted by the claimants.

9. Claimants retain legal representation immediately after the accident is reported.

---

[2] INSURANCE FRAUD: HANDBOOK FOR INSURANCE PERSONNEL, National Insurance Crime Bureau (1999)

10. Past experience demonstrates that the physician's bill and report, regardless of the varying accident circumstances, are always the same.

11. Treatment prescribed for various injuries resulting from differing accidents is always the same in terms of duration and type of therapy.

12. Medical bills indicate routine treatment being provided on Sundays or holidays.

13. Treatment for extensive injuries is protracted, even though the accident was minor.

14. Worker's compensation insurer and health carrier are billed simultaneously; payment is accepted from both.

15. Injured worker protests about returning to work and never seems to improve.

16. Summary medical bills are submitted without dates or descriptions of office visits.

17. Medical bills submitted are photocopies of originals.

18. Extensive or unnecessary treatment for minor, subjective injuries.

Some of the above indicators, by themselves, are not necessarily suspicious. But several indicators together become something that is important for chiropractors to watch out for. When three new patients involved in the same accident arrive on the same day the accident occurred, all complaining of vague neck and back pain that is given at 9/10, who already have legal representation, such a case should raise your suspicions.

Straw Owners

New York State requires medical clinics to be fully owned, operated, and controlled by licensed physicians, and proof of such physician ownership needs to be furnished to an insurer along with a claim (block 17 of the NF-3; see Appendix C). By law, claims for services from clinics that are not actively owned by a physician are not eligible for reimbursement. Since many no-fault mills are not actually owned and managed by licensed physicians, the only way mill owners can appear to satisfy this legal requirement is to recruit physicians to act as straw owners. A straw owner physician will be paid by the mill owners to sign the PC incorporation paperwork and bank documents, but the P.C.'s bank account will actually be controlled by the mill owners. These physicians may receive their payment in the form of an inflated salary that does not correlate with their duties or hours worked.

Prosecutors in cases of fraud are given broad leeway to assess a physician's actual ownership of a P.C.; in a landmark 2005 decision,[3] the New York State Court of Appeals held that investigators may "look beyond the face" of documents to corroborate fraud. Prosecutors and investigators may consider whether the purported physician-owner has actual control of the P.C. and incurs any risk of economic loss. This decision was recently upheld in another case,[4] where a physician straw owner argued, unsuccessfully, that she was the actual owner and that ownership should be defined only formally (by whose name appears on the incorporation documents).

This has serious implications for chiropractors who join a clinic controlled by others. A clinic owner may tell you, as a chiropractor, that he will rent you a treatment room in his

---

[3] State Farm Mut. Auto Ins. Co. v. Mallela, 4 N,Y.3d 313 (2005)

[4] United States v. Gabinskaya, Docket No.15-776-cr

high-volume no-fault clinic, and will even helpfully set up a P.C. for you. He may also generously offer (or insist, as part of the terms) to do your billing and collections for you—for a nominal fee, of course, included in the monthly rent, which he will take right off the top and give you the rest, depositing it directly into the P.C.'s account for you. He will assure you that you will, of course, receive all the insurance statements too, so you can see that everything is aboveboard.

Sounds reasonable, maybe? Well, guess what—under such an arrangement, you would be a straw owner because it has all the essential elements necessary for prosecutors to consider it as such. What the clinic owner is really doing is paying you to set up a P.C. in your name which he controls and bills under, while taking a big cut of your collections for the privilege of you having access to "his" patients.

Such arrangements are quite prevalent in the no-fault world, but that doesn't make them legal or ethical. Any chiropractor considering such an arrangement should be very afraid, and any chiropractor already involved in such an arrangement should start looking to get away from it.

> *Ironically, during the writing of this chapter a friend of mine who is a physical medicine physician called me to tell me about an "opportunity" she had just been offered. A young businessman, "Alex,", was starting a mobile testing business, performing electrodiagnostic tests (NCV & EMG). He had many accounts in no-fault clinics, and he needed an MD experienced in electrodiagnostics to interpret the studies and occasionally perform EMGs—for which he was offering a generous salary. What he also wanted, however, was for my physician friend to "hold the P.C." for the testing company (remember, because only claims for medical services from entities wholly owned*

and controlled by physicians are eligible for reimbursement). The billing was all going to be done through a law firm that "Alex" had an arrangement with. "Alex" also told her that she may have to go to an EUO every few months. (EUO, or Examination Under Oath, is an investigative process similar to a deposition, where an attorney or investigator for the insurance company interrogates the provider, the claimant, or both, regarding details of the accident or injuries in order to determine the veracity of the claim). Not only was my friend uncomfortable with the obvious straw-owner proposal, the prospect of potentially having to lie about it at an EUO made it even worse. Needless to say, she turned down "Alex's" offer.

This kind of unsolicited anecdote underscores just how prevalent such illegal business arrangements are, and how important it is for chiropractors (and anyone else) to do their due diligence in ensuring that there isn't even the appearance of impropriety in their business and professional relationships.

Unperformed Services

Mill-type clinics frequently bill for services that have not actually been performed. Not just for fake visits—although as we will see, that also happens—but more along the lines of including unperformed services along with services that were actually performed in a visit.

In chiropractic, this can take the form of upcoding, which is billing for a level of service higher (and more expensive) than the one actually performed. For example, coding for a complex and detailed history and initial examination when only a problem-focused examination was performed. Many doctors don't necessarily think of this as billing for an unperformed service; after all, an examination was done, wasn't it? Well, yes. But the one billed for wasn't, and *that's* the unperformed service. Do enough of these, and you can land in pretty big trouble—especially if there are other improprieties associated with your practice.

Another form of unperformed service is known as "unbundling." This refers to separately billing for different procedures that are normally considered part of the same service, for higher reimbursement. In no-fault, this never used to be a big issue with chiropractic, because for a long time there really wasn't much to unbundle. Chiropractic visits were reimbursed at a flat global fee regardless of how many actual services were performed, with a single procedure code used (usually 99213). However, in December 2010 the chiropractic fee schedule changed to an RVU-based system, where chiropractors could bill different procedures separately to a limit of 8 RVUs per day. Suddenly, it became possible to collect more per visit by billing certain codes together, which of course, many chiropractors saw as an invitation to do just that—even when the services were already bundled or may have been unnecessary.

As a practical example of such unbundling, in most no-fault clinics chiropractors generally don't apply any physiotherapy modalities (heat, electrical muscle stimulation, ultrasound) to patients, because that's what the clinic's physical therapists do; the chiropractor "just adjusts" (and does initial and reexaminations). A spinal adjustment alone is either 4.57 RVUs (98940) or 6 RVUs (98941), leaving 2-3 RVUs on the table (98942 is usually not frequently used). Since passive modalities are already done by the PT, chiropractors add more active treatment codes, such as massage (97124, 2.62 RVUs), therapeutic exercises (97110, 3.97 RVUs) or neuromuscular re-education (97112, 3.89 RVUs). These combinations are fine when the services are necessary, indicated, and documented. The problem is, they are often not . . . and billing them is unperformed services—in other words, fraud.

Even when they are indicated, some procedures cannot be performed on the same area that is also adjusted—for example, you can't adjust the lumbar spine and then bill for 15 minutes of massage to the lumbar spine because soft tissue work is considered part of the adjustment service. The same with an unspecified procedure like "manual therapy"—that too, cannot be billed when performed on an area that was also adjusted. What I did when I had my own practice is when a patient had a lumbar complaint, I would always assess for hamstring tightness. The hamstrings can affect the lumbar spine since they attach to the pelvis, and hypertonic hamstring muscles can exert tension on the pelvis, in turn stressing the lumbar spine and affecting proper function. Many people have overly tight hamstrings, and stretching them (properly, for a minimum of 8 minutes combined) can positively augment the adjustment to the lumbar spine, while being a separate area from it. That is how to properly bill for another procedure, without unbundling.

> *I once covered a clinic in a gritty part of Queens for a couple of days, and I quickly suspected that it was probably a "mill." It was a very large facility, with at least twelve curtained physical therapy "bays" on one end and a bank of examination rooms on the other. The chiropractic treatment area was one of those pictured earlier in this book—a bench table stuck into a corner behind a curtain.*
>
> *"Dr. Sergey", the chiropractor who had hired me, wanted to meet with me briefly on the first day to "go over the notes." As in many clinics, the daily notes were a check-off format: a sheet for every patient with four or five visit blocks, each with symptoms, objective*

findings, and procedure codes to check-off for that visit. The sheets were kept in a three-ring binder and alphabetized by the patient's last name.

As he showed me the binder, he pointed to the sheets (which I had seen before, since many clinics use the same type of sheet) and said, "make sure you put for every patient [an] adjustment and either 97110 (therapeutic exercises) or 97112 (neuromuscular re-education)."

I had encountered these kinds of instructions once before while doing coverage. Note that there were two things wrong with his instructions: one, the fact that I was asked to do this for every patient—not just the ones for whom it might have been necessary; and two, I wasn't asked to actually do the procedures—I was asked only to "put" the billing code for them.

Obviously, I wasn't going to follow such directions. I certainly wasn't going to indicate that I had performed a procedure that I hadn't. What I could, and did do, was assessed which patients had an indication for those procedures, and then actually do them with the patients. Not every patient had an indication—some were too acute. But I was able to do some active post-isometric relaxation exercises, hamstring stretches, pelvic tilts and bridges, and exercise ball techniques with some patients, for the required minimum amount of time (8 minutes). Of course, I manually documented the procedures and the indication for them in the small place on the sheet for handwritten notes.

What was remarkable, although not entirely unexpected, was that when I was doing these techniques with the patients, they all acted as if this was something unusual—because it was. I asked *patients if any of the other chiropractors who treated them had done anything like this, or even remotely similar, and they all said no. Of course they didn't; neuromuscular re-education and therapeutic exercise are active, direct-contact, timed (15-minute) procedures that require a minimum of 8 minutes of procedure time. And that's in addition to the time it takes to adjust a patient. It's not physically possible to do them on every patient when you're seeing 45–50 patients per ten-hour day.*

I never worked for that doctor again. But I am sure that this was not an isolated practice. Insurance companies are vigilant for these things, though, and their SIUs (Special Investigative Units) are trained to detect these kinds of billing patterns. Not all fraud gets detected, but some does, and if the authorities get involved, which they sometimes do, the consequences can be devastating. It's not worth it.

Claimant and Patient Fraud

Sometimes, the patients themselves may be actively involved in fraud. It doesn't happen often, but occasionally a patient may be brazen (or stupid) enough to openly suggest that you commit fraud or to assist them in doing so. You should feel very comfortable showing these patients the door.

Early in my career, I was working full-time in a relatively decent no-fault clinic when the office manager at the front desk called me in my office. "There's a new patient here, but he wants to speak to you first before he fills out any paperwork."

I told her to send him on back, and a lanky man walked in and sat in the chair by my desk. I asked him what he wanted to speak to me about.

"Well, doc, first I just wanna say that I get all my treatment over by the Medical Center," he said, referring to a large local county hospital. "But what I wanna do wit' you is, I wanna come in here, sign my name on the sheet, and then you give me half of what you charge."

I stared at him incredulously. He was openly proposing to sign his name on my sheet (and whatever else), and then have me submit bills for services never performed, which would be split with him for the "privilege." "I . . . can't do that," I said, chuckling slightly.

"Ok, doc, that's fine . . . I'll jus' find someone else, then," he said. I politely showed him the door. Then I called his referring attorney and informed him what a fine upstanding human being his (hopefully soon-to-be former) client was.

Much later in my career I was working in another clinic, and there was a patient who had come in as part of a group of three who were in the same accident. I only saw two of them, since the third had no spinal complaints at the time. They were rather urban, even thuggy-looking individuals, who no doubt had more than a passing acquaintance with the criminal justice system, and the tattoos to prove it.

One day, one that had always given me a particularly weird vibe came into the room and signed his name on the sign-in sheet. "I don't wanna get my back cracked today."

"Okay," I said. "We can do something else—what do you want to do?"

"Nothin, man," he replied. "I wanna go home . . . I'm tired." (It was about 11:30 AM.)

I told him that he was welcome to skip the visit, but that he couldn't expect to just sign his name (as if he received treatment) and leave. "Why not? He sneered. "Ain't no cameras in here. You gon' snitch?"

I informed him that we wouldn't be submitting any visits that weren't actually performed, and he decided to stay that day after all. But I decided that going forward, the best course of action in this case would be to discharge him from my care and allow him to just keep getting physical therapy. I informed the office staff and the medical director about the incident and they were all in agreement with my decision.

4

INSURANCE INDUSTRY RESPONSE

Fraud and overutilization have not gone unnoticed by automobile insurance companies, though some chiropractors might like to believe that they have. In late 2010, the Insurance Research Council conducted an industry-wide study of over 4,500 New York no-fault claims from among over ten different insurers—including GEICO, Allstate, Progressive, State Farm, and others. Their findings indicated that no-fault fraud in New York is on the rise, and continuing to do so.[5]

Injury claims payment amounts jumped an average of 52% between 2005 and 2010, with those increases mainly coming from the downstate region (NYC metropolitan area).

---

[5] Neis, Al. "No-Fault NY: Is It As Good As Advertised?" Buckeye Actuarial Continuing Education, April 2011. PowerPoint Presentation.

The researchers found that more claimants from the downstate region had similar injury patterns, visited pain clinics and larger numbers of providers, received more diagnostic tests and durable medical equipment, and were more likely to hire an attorney than claimants from the upstate region. The report concluded that while there are other possible reasons for this disparity, a major reason is fraud and "buildup" of cases. The No-Fault Unit of the New York State Department of Financial Services, Frauds Bureau, reported an almost 10% increase in no-fault fraud between 2006 (10117 cases) and 2009 (13,433 cases). In 2015, the most recent year available, of 22,762 fraud reports received from insurers, 12,891 (57%) were for suspected no-fault fraud.

The report also compared treatment trends between the upstate and downstate regions. More downstate claimants than upstate saw a chiropractor (49% vs. 21%), a physical therapist (42% vs. 18%), an acupuncturist 34% vs. 7%) and a pain specialist (23% vs. 8%). More claimants from the New York City area received MRIs than their upstate counterparts (50% vs. 20%), and more EMG studies (24% vs. 4%). More claimants in NYC saw a PT and DC in combination than upstate (32% vs. 7%), and almost half of the downstate claimants saw more than 4 different providers in a multidisciplinary clinic than the rest of the state (44% vs. 12-14%).

(An interesting treatment trend the researchers found was that while patients were more likely to have had more than 50 visits to a physical therapist in NYC than upstate (18% vs. 10%), about the same number of patients saw a chiropractor more than 50 times in *both* areas—about 20%. While this data could be interpreted to mean that there is chiropractic overutilization in both areas, it could also be interpreted as 20% of chiropractic no-fault patients requiring more treatment, especially when considered against the other comparative treatment data. I believe that this is actually more likely.)

By law, insurers in New York State must have special investigation units (SIUs) to investigate suspect claims (although as mentioned earlier, the thirty-day rule often prevents a comprehensive investigation before the claim must be paid or denied). Insurers may also refer certain suspect claims, referred to as "questionable claims" (QC), where there is suspected organized crime or gang activity (OGAs), to the National Insurance Crime Bureau to assist their SIUs to more thoroughly investigate. According to a 2012 report, the NICB was referred over 13,000 QC/OGAs by insurers, with New York being in the top 5 referring states and the #2 referring city; the most common reason for a QC/OGA was a suspected staged accident.

Of course, all insurance companies analyze policy and claims data extensively in determining whether a particular claim is suspicious. In addition to the indicators enumerated earlier, some other "red flags" that an SIU investigator might look for are different policies purchased from the same computer, email address, or IP address—which means that insurance companies can tell where you are! -—and this data is being logged and mined. They also look for the same individual requesting multiple quotes, for multiple drivers, multiple vehicles, or a combination of these. A big red flag is when an initial premium payment check bounces on a new policy—that triggers an alert that an accident claim may be imminent.

So what are insurance companies doing about fraud? One measure being taken is pushing for legislative reform. Earlier, we mentioned S424—the anti-runner bill. There is another bill in the New York State Legislature, S2816A, that proposes broad reforms in the insurance laws to tighten the gaps that make it easier to commit the kinds of fraud plaguing the industry and consumers alike. Some of the proposed changes to the law include:

- Defining "health service provider."

- Loosening the provisions of the "thirty-day rule" that mandate payment of non-meritorious claims, so as to make it more feasible for insurers to conduct claims investigations; the bill would also require more burden of proof on the claimant and the provider to show necessity, rather than the burden being on the insurer to refute the claim. Currently, only a medical bill is required to establish a claim.

- Requiring mandatory arbitration for no-fault disputes rather than litigation, often for small amounts, that drags the claims process out 4-5 times longer. Recall that the entire point of the no-fault laws was reducing congestion in the courts and the time to get reimbursed.

- Amending the no-fault assignment of benefits to remove the right of medical providers to contest policy, coverage and eligibility issues on the claimant's behalf. Current law allows providers to contest such issues, which results in a lot of litigation caused by the provider, independently of the claimant. It would also invalidate the assignment when there is any dispute regarding policy compliance or coverage being in effect.

- Making it less difficult to decertify certain providers from billing or collecting payments from no-fault insurance.

- Establishing rigorous treatment guidelines, including authorizations, such as are already in effect within the Worker's Compensation system. This will greatly reduce overutilization and billing over fee schedule. (It will also greatly negatively impact patient care, in my opinion. In my experience, the Worker's Comp system is a terrible system to try and get anything done for a patient, and has created its own industry of lawyers that exist to fight it; instituting treatment guidelines that are too restrictive will only be trading one set of problems for another.)

- Allow an insurer to cancel a policy or revoke coverage within the first 60 days for nonpayment of premium or where a policy was fraudulently obtained.

As of this writing, Bill S2816A has passed both the New York Senate and Assembly and is awaiting delivery to the Governor. As with S424, it remains to be seen whether this bill will be passed into law, revised, or vetoed.

NO-FAULT WITH NO FEAR

5

LEGAL RAMIFICATIONS

Previously, we discussed different ways fraud typically occurs, and how insurers deal with cases of suspected fraud. When suspicion is high enough and enough supporting data has been gathered, cases are turned over to the police, the State Attorney General's or District Attorney's office, or to the district office of the U.S. Justice Department. Investigators (detectives or Federal agents) then take over the investigation and gather evidence, sometimes for months or years, that leads to the arrest of suspects. It is instructive to review some of the relevant laws concerning fraud and other related offenses because knowing the elements of an offense can be essential in being able to recognize and avoid illegal activity.

Overview of Relevant Laws

Although not an exhaustive and comprehensive list of offenses, there are several relevant statutes that are usually applied, often in combination, when prosecuting no-fault fraud. Among them are: at the State level, Grand Larceny, Insurance Fraud, Enterprise Corruption, Conspiracy, and Falsifying Business Records. At the Federal level, the most common statutes applied to no-fault fraud are Health Care Fraud and Conspiracy, as well as Mail & Wire Fraud and Money Laundering.

Grand Larceny (NYPL 155.30-155.42)

In New York State, theft in any form of money or property valued at over one thousand dollars constitutes Grand Larceny. The degree, and corresponding felony level and sentencing range, depends on how much money or value is involved. Grand Larceny in the fourth degree (E Felony) involves amounts in excess of $1,000; third degree (D Felony), in excess of $3,000; second degree (C Felony) in excess of $50,000; and first degree (B Felony) is for amounts over $1 million. Sentencing ranges are up to 4, 7, 15, and 25 years in prison, respectively.

Insurance Fraud (NYPL 176.00-176.35)

All insurance fraud must incorporate what is called a "fraudulent act" as defined in the statute, which can include altering written documents, concealing, falsifying, misrepresenting or deleting information that will be presented to or by an insurer. This definition can obviously include things like chiropractic treatment notes, billing and diagnosis codes (remember upcoding and unbundling?), dates, and the actual provider of treatment. Regardless of any monetary loss or gain, the "fraudulent act" is by itself insurance fraud in the fifth degree and is a class A misdemeanor. As with Grand Larceny, degrees four through first degree, and their felony levels and penalty ranges, are dependent on the monetary amount involved. Insurance

Fraud in the fourth degree (E Felony) involves amounts in excess of $1,000; third degree (D Felony), in excess of $3,000; second degree (C Felony) in excess of $50,000; and first degree (B Felony) is for amounts over $1 million. Sentencing ranges again are up to 4, 7, 15, and 25 years in prison, respectively.

Falsifying Business Records (NYPL 175.05 (1-4)

Making changes to business or financial records that is also related to, aids in, or is intended to conceal another crime is Felony Falsification of Business Records, an E Felony. Straw owners and others who pay inflated rents and fees to clinic owners for "billing services" that are really just disguised fee-splitting could be charged under this statute (along with others).

Enterprise Corruption (NYPL 460.20)

This is a complex statute that is a powerful tool of prosecutors, often brought in large cases where there is an association between insurance fraud and/or larceny to a criminal organization—say, a network of clinic owners that also have ties to other criminal activity. Charges of Enterprise Corruption may be brought when there is a pattern of criminal activity with knowing participation in the organization's affairs, if one invests in its proceeds, or has an interest in the organization. In theory, if a chiropractor is involved with owners of several clinics, who are also involved with other illegal activities (such as laundering the clinics' proceeds), this could be considered involvement with a criminal enterprise. Enterprise Corruption carries a penalty of up to 25 years in prison.

Conspiracy (NYPL 105.00-105.35)

Generally speaking, Conspiracy means that at least two persons agree to engage in criminal conduct, and one of those persons commits an "overt act" in the furtherance of the conspiracy. The degree of the conspiracy offense (at the State level) depends on the type and degree of the offense being conspired to commit.

Importantly, according to the statute, "unawareness of the criminal nature of the agreement or the object conduct or of the defendant's criminal purpose" is, among other things, not a defense; in other words, "not knowing what other people were going to do, or that what was going on was wrong" doesn't matter. It also doesn't matter if the "overt act" that furthered the conspiracy was itself illegal or not—only that it furthered the conspiracy. (The Federal conspiracy statute is similar, as we will see.) This makes Conspiracy one of the most powerful tools a prosecutor has—it can be molded to include almost any conduct that relates to an offense.

Federal Statutes

In prosecuting cases of no-fault fraud, sometimes Federal charges are brought by the U.S. Justice Department, especially if the case is large enough. Below are some of the Federal statutes that are often applied to the prosecution of no-fault fraud:

Mail Fraud & Wire Fraud (18 USC 1341, 1343)

Mail Fraud is one of the most frequently brought charges in so-called "white-collar" cases, such as health, financial, or insurance schemes; along with Wire Fraud (18 USC 1343), it can be tailored to fit almost any type of conduct associated with an offense. Essentially, using the mail (or UPS or FedEx), or a telephone (or a fax, or the internet) during the course of a fraudulent scheme can meet the criteria for these charges—even if the mail or phone use was not itself of an illegal or criminal nature—as long as it was used in the course of the fraud.

Health Care Fraud (18 USC 1347)

Health Care Fraud was enacted as a statute in 1996 in response to soaring healthcare costs. Since the Federal government is the largest spender of health care dollars in the United States, it has tried to control costs through all possible means, including aggressively pursuing health care fraud. The statute itself is not terribly long, and bears citing in full here:

```
18 U.S. Code § 1347 —Health care fraud

(a) Whoever knowingly and willfully
executes, or attempts to execute, a
scheme or artifice—
(1) to defraud any health care benefit
program; or
(2) to obtain, by means of false or
fraudulent pretenses, representations, or
promises, any of the money or property
owned by, or under the custody or control
of, any health care benefit program, in
connection with the delivery of or
payment for health care benefits, items,
or services, shall be fined under this
title or imprisoned not more than 10
years, or both. If the violation results
in serious bodily injury (as defined in
section 1365 of this title), such person
```

```
shall be fined under this title or
imprisoned not more than 20 years, or
both; and if the violation results in
death, such person shall be fined under
this title, or imprisoned for any term of
years or for life, or both.
(b) With respect to violations of this
section, a person need not have actual
knowledge of this section or specific
intent to commit a violation of this
section.
```

Note the last paragraph: no specific intent to commit a crime is necessary to be guilty. As with many Federal crimes, only the barest elements need be present for prosecutors to be able to bring charges. But 18 USC 1347—unlike the statutes for Mail and Wire Fraud—obviates even the requirement of intent to break the law.

Conspiracy

Finally, we come to probably the most fearsome charge Federal prosecutors can wield—Conspiracy. Many people erroneously believe that conspiracy is a conscious process, that two or more people need to sit down and spell out the crime they intend to commit, and formally "agree" on it. However, the elements of conspiracy are quite broad. As with the State conspiracy statute, the offense necessitates that at least two or more persons "agree" to commit a crime, such as Health Care Fraud. As mentioned before, one need not have specific intent to commit a crime—or even consciously be aware of an "agreement"—the conspiracy exists independently of the conspirators' awareness of it as such. All that is required is that they agree to further the conspiracy. This agreement can be implied.

Additionally, one of the conspirators must commit an "overt act" that furthers the conspiracy; but that overt act need not be illegal or criminal, and the other conspirators don't need to know about it. The conspirators need not even be aware of all the other conspirators. **The government must only prove negligence; that a person was aware of—or *should* have been aware of—a common criminal purpose, and was a willing participant.** It's not even necessary for the crime being conspired to be successful, or even attempted; conspiracy is a crime in and of itself.

If that doesn't chill you to the core, it should. Using the barest details, a prosecutor can charge conspiracy for just about anything. In fact, conspiracy charges are among Federal prosecutors' favorites and are often used to leverage a plea bargain and get defendants to provide information and cooperation against other defendants in the case. And the kicker is that the penalties for conspiracy are the same as for the overt offense—in other words, conspiracy to commit health care fraud carries the same 10-year maximum sentence as does actual health care fraud; it's the government's "in for a penny, in for a pound" doctrine on conspiracy.

Prosecutors are given wide discretion when it comes to looking at the circumstances of a situation and deciding whether to bring charges, what charges to bring, and against whom to bring them. Something that may seem like it should be a civil or administrative issue can easily be criminalized by a prosecutor who decides there's enough evidence to build a criminal case, especially if he or she wants cooperation against a "bigger fish". It's not worth being even minimally involved with criminal activity because as we will see, the penalties for being on the wrong side of that prosecutorial discretion can be draconian.

Implications for Chiropractors

So what does this all mean for chiropractors?

As I've said before, no-fault practice is a very large part of chiropractic in New York, at least in the metropolitan region, and if the no-fault system were to suddenly exclude chiropractic, half the profession in NY (or more) would probably quickly disappear.

While that's not likely to happen, the current system has been exploited and abused and is not sustainable in the long term. Thirty years ago, when someone was involved in a car accident, they went to see their medical doctor, who would refer them for physical therapy. Or they might have gone to see their chiropractor, who would adjust them and also do physiotherapy modalities with them. Sending a patient to a pain specialist or for special testing like EMG meant referring the patient out. The patient had to "leave the house" and go to that specialist's office—inconvenient for the patient and distasteful for many chiropractors, who at that time were never quite sure how a medical specialist might view them. This meant that if you were going to refer a patient out, it was probably going to be because you really thought the test or consult was necessary, and not because it was part of the conveyor belt of specialists. Fraud has always been around, yes; our friend Hegestratos will attest to that. But the advent of multidisciplinary accident clinics, while convenient for patients and certainly not without merit, has also created incentives for overutilization and fraud.

No-fault clinics abound in the NYC metropolitan area. An informal survey of a popular chiropractic employment web page revealed 166 job postings within a three-month period; of the 161 non-academic job opportunities posted, 25 jobs were upstate (Westchester & Rockland counties and above), with only a single one for a no-fault clinic. Of the remaining

136 downstate jobs, exactly 50% (68) were for no-fault clinics.[6]

With so many no-fault clinics, and so many cases of fraud and questionable claims reported, it's unlikely that a chiropractor who has spent time working in such clinics has not been exposed to fraud in some way. If you have a P.C. with space in a clinic, and you are not completely autonomous (i.e., you do not completely control your billing, clinical decision-making, treatment plans and frequency, etc.), then it is very possible that you are involved with a fraudulent enterprise. The same is true if you are an employee working for another chiropractor who fits those criteria; simply following instructions does not necessarily shield you from responsibility.

On the other hand, one has to work and pay bills. With half the available employment opportunities in the area being in no-fault clinics, eschewing them is not really a practical option. Besides, as we discussed, there is definite merit to multidisciplinary clinics. Therefore, the best thing a doctor of chiropractic can—and should—do, is to be extremely careful. Be vigilant for the signs of fraud, know who you're getting involved with, what the operational details are (as much as possible), and be prepared to walk away if you feel uncomfortable. No job, no business opportunity is worth sacrificing your professional ethics (or worse, risking prosecution). It's not necessary to become an investigator; that's what insurance companies have SIUs for. Especially as an employee doctor, you're not required to know the source of every patient referral or reconstruct their accident; if a patient

---

[6] No-fault clinics were identified by the presence of at least two of the following indicators: use of the words "no fault," "multidisciplinary," or "high volume" in the ad text, the author's familiarity with the employer's clinic as being no-fault, and hours and location of job being highly consistent with those of a typical no-fault clinic. Postings mentioning Medicare, family practice, sports rehab, nutrition, wellness, "holistic," or specifically excluding no-fault were not considered.

has been in an accident and complains to you of pain, you must take them at their word, but also confirm it with objective findings.

Sadly, some chiropractors fail to heed this advice, with disastrous results. In the next chapter, we will examine two real cases where chiropractors might have saved themselves a world of trouble if they had only been more conscientious.

6

CASE STUDIES IN FRAUD

We've seen how the laws we discussed can theoretically be applied to fraudulent activity. Here we will examine how those laws were actually applied in real state and Federal criminal cases, where chiropractors were unfortunately involved.

The Zemlyansky Case

Mikhail "Russian Mike" Zemlyansky was, according to his neighbors in Hewlett, Long Island, a nice guy who "had a business." But they never knew that his business was fraud.

Zemlyansky, who was also something of a semi-professional gambler (he won $75,000 in a 2009 poker tournament at the Borgata in Atlantic City, where he was a regular), owned and controlled dozens of no-fault clinics across the metropolitan area together with his partner, a man named Michael Danilovich, and others. And they used those clinics to print money.

The general idea was simple: get accident victims as patients and bill the dickens out of the insurance. To that end, Zemlyansky and Danilovich created an elaborate network of clinics and controllers and recruited doctors as straw owners. Two of the straw doctors, Sergey Gabinsky and Tatyana Gabinskaya, were paid $10,000 a month to set up clinic P.C.s and business accounts in their names and sign clinic paperwork for Zemlyansky and Danilovich. Runners were paid $2000-3,000 to recruit the patients, who were then also paid $500. The patients were also referred to attorneys, who paid the two Mikes $1,000 per referral. The clinics billed out hundreds of millions of dollars in medical, chiropractic, acupuncture, and other treatments, as well as various tests, durable medical equipment, and other services.

The money that poured in was then carefully laundered through various shell companies—some in Eastern Europe—by writing blank checks for just under $10,000 (a "structured" amount to avoid bank's reporting requirements of deposits exceeding $10,000). These checks would be given to "cashers" who would cash the checks and bring back the cash to be distributed and used to pay all the kickbacks to and from the controllers, as well as to pay the runners and the patients. Some insurance payments went into the straw P.C. accounts, from which checks would be written to other dummy companies as "expenses", and then Zemlyansky and Danilovich would pay their personal expenses from the dummy company accounts.

Sometime in the middle of 2010, the insurer GEICO got suspicious, and together with the NICB, began an investigation. They contacted the authorities, who set up telephone wiretaps and sent in two undercover NYPD detectives to pose as patients. The undercover patients collected evidence for months, coming in for "treatment" which they sometimes did not have. According to then- Police Commissioner Ray Kelly, when they were directed to the chiropractor's office, they were told to "sign in, say hello, and leave." They were paid for coming in as well.

The Chiropractors

Chad Greenshner and Constantine Voytenko were two chiropractors who were affiliated with Zemlyansky's clinics. Zemlyansky and Danilovich controlled at least 15 different clinics; one of Voytenko's was a tidy storefront on a side street in the Sheepshead Bay area of Brooklyn, sandwiched between a TD Bank and a two-family house. An awning sign announced its rather nondescript name of "Medical Plaza, P.C.." Investigators say that clinics like that one often saw up to 150 people come through in one day. It's not spelled out in any documents, but the likelihood is that Greenshner and Voytenko were the two chiropractic P.C. holders for all the clinics, and hired other chiropractors to work in them. It's entirely possible that Greenshner and Voytenko never themselves saw a single patient in any of the clinics.

On February 29, 2012, Zemlyansky, Danilovich, Greenshner, and Voytenko, along with Gabinsky and Gabinskaya, eight other physicians, two acupuncturists, three attorneys, and seventeen other individuals were arrested in the early morning by FBI agents. The U.S. Attorney for the Eastern District at the time, Preet Bharara, called it the biggest no-fault fraud bust in history—$279 million. The chiropractors were both charged with one count each of Conspiracy to commit Health Care Fraud and Conspiracy to commit Mail Fraud.

We can speculate about the others, but what were the chiropractors thinking? Greenshner and Voytenko were nice, otherwise good people. Voytenko was a children's swimming coach. Greenshner once helped give first aid to an injured woman whose car was hit by a falling crane.[7] Did they enter this arrangement consciously intending to commit fraud? Or did they think they were just smart businessmen, doing what all the other chiropractors in the industry were doing—renting some space in busy clinics and farming out associates to see patients who were in legitimate accidents?

Unfortunately, it doesn't matter what their intentions were. Remember conspiracy? Prosecutors can tease any thread of detail in a case and weave it into a conspiracy charge. There's no need for specific intent to commit a crime; there's no need to spell out a plan among conspirators. There's not even a need for the crime to be successful. All that's legally necessary is to be involved and to have been able to know that some part of the process was illegal. Those are pretty wide criteria—you could drive a truck through them. Even if the accidents were legitimate (which, according to investigators, they were)—and even if their employee chiropractors were treating their patients appropriately (and there's no reason to think they weren't, since Greenshner and Voytenko were the only chiropractors charged)—the entire organization was tainted. Their partners were crooked, the business structure was fraudulent, everything about the clinics was fraudulent—and so the treatments were considered excessive and unnecessary.

Greenshner and Voytenko each pleaded guilty to one count of 18 USC 1349—Conspiracy to Commit Health Care Fraud. Greenshner served six months in Federal prison. Voytenko received three years' probation. Both lost their licenses.

The moral of the story is to make certain that not only do you do everything legally and properly but that you do not get

---

[7] September 30, 2006, "Five injured in partial crane collapse." Originally aired on WABC-NY, 7 Online; retrieved from: http://www.ufanyc.org/cms/contents/view/3748

involved with parties who may be doing anything improper. If you don't know, ask, and verify the answers as much as possible. If you don't get answers (or if you get the wrong ones), you may need to rethink your involvement.

And what about the two Mikes—Zemlyansky and Danilovich? Well, they gave the Feds a good fight—after all, they had money to pay the best lawyers. Zemlyansky was offered a plea deal for a maximum of ten years, but incredibly, turned it down. He went to trial, twice—the first time, in 2013, he won a mistrial on one count and an acquittal on eight others, but the government took him to trial again on the rest. The second time, in March 2015, Zemlyansky was convicted of racketeering conspiracy, securities fraud, wire fraud, and mail fraud after a four-week trial. He was sentenced to 15 years in Federal prison.

Danilovich also went to trial twice. The first time, in 2013, a unanimous verdict could not be reached, and the trial ended in a hung jury. But the Feds never give up, and after another five-week trial in 2016, Danilovich was finally convicted of 16 counts of racketeering conspiracy, securities fraud, health care fraud, mail fraud, wire fraud, and money laundering. He was sentenced to 25 years in Federal prison. He will be 64 years old when he is released.

The Vinarsky Case

Gregory Vinarsky was the manager of several clinics in upper Manhattan in the mid to late 2000's. He basically ran the show—hired the staff and doctors, ordered supplies, and made sure everyone got the services he wanted them to get—whether they were necessary or not.

Vinarsky employed a medical physician, Aron Goldman, and also had a chiropractor, Matthew Keschner, seeing the patients in his facilities. There were several other MDs, as well as acupuncturists and physical therapists employed as well, as is typical of no-fault clinics.

Vinarsky was basically doing everything wrong that we discussed in earlier chapters—he was paying runners, staging accidents, coaching patients, employing straw owners, splitting fees, and rendering unnecessary services. He was the director in every sense of the word, and the doctors and therapists in his clinic were merely functioning as willing cogs in his massive fraud machine. Keschner didn't direct any clinic affairs, and wasn't himself a straw owner, and did not seem to be involved in recruiting patients. Nevertheless, he was named as a principal defendant in the case.

A comprehensive description of the details of this case comes from New York State Court of Appeals Judge Eugene Fahey, in his opinion[8] upholding chiropractor Matthew Keschner's conviction of Enterprise Corruption. It is excerpted below, with emphasis added to highlight issues discussed previously in this and other chapters, and footnoted with my comments.

I.

Defendant Matthew Keschner was a licensed chiropractor. Defendant Aron Goldman was licensed to practice medicine. They began working in 2001 at a medical clinic in Manhattan started by Gregory Vinarsky. Vinarsky employed "runners" who listened to police scanners to learn where car accidents had occurred and then **approached the accident victims and offered to pay them to go to the clinic**. Vinarsky then referred the patients to certain lawyers, who **paid kickbacks to him for the referrals. He established**

---

[8] People v Keschner 2015 NY Slip Op 05596. Decided on June 30, 2015 Court of Appeals; Fahey, J. Published by New York State Law Reporting Bureau pursuant to Judiciary Law § 431

relationships with managers of facilities that carried out tests such as MRIs and X rays, who made payments to his clinic in exchange for referrals. He also arranged to receive kickbacks from companies from which durable medical equipment could be ordered.[9] **At the clinic, Vinarsky ensured that personnel prescribed the maximum number of tests, treatments, and items of medical equipment that no-fault insurance would cover, regardless of a patient's need.**

Goldman was listed as the owner of the clinic on incorporation papers. New York requires that the owner of an incorporated medical clinic be licensed to practice medicine, and Vinarsky was not licensed. Keschner incorporated his chiropractic practice under his own name. Goldman, an internist, was on a salary, while **Vinarsky's arrangement with Keschner was profit-sharing in exchange for referrals.**[10] Vinarsky also had similar referral arrangements with an acupuncturist and a neurologist. In 2002, Vinarsky shut this clinic down, and opened another, St. Nicholas Medical Clinic, near Columbia University Medical Center, running the same scheme with the same personnel. Vinarsky selected the location of the new clinic, chose its employees, ordered medical supplies, hired and managed the "runners," and oversaw the paperwork and billing submitted to the insurance companies. **He also opened bank accounts and created management companies into which proceeds were placed. Goldman again became a salaried employee at the clinic, and was named as the owner on incorporation documents.**[11] He

---

[9] All textbook examples of illegal fee-splitting and kickbacks.

[10] Another classic example of fee-splitting. All arrangements should be straight rental only and based on market rates, not contingent on percent of profits.

[11] A classic straw-ownership scenario.

worked at the clinic three days a week. **Vinarsky and Keschner again had a profit-sharing arrangement; Keschner kept 35% of the profits his chiropractic corporation generated, and gave the rest to Vinarsky.** Keschner worked three days a week, and **hired a second chiropractor to assist him**.[12] Vinarsky, meanwhile, hired two physicians to supplement Goldman.

Vinarsky created a preprinted initial evaluation form that the doctors at the clinic completed for each patient. **The first entry in its "Treatment Plan" template, for example, was "The patient advised to attend a supervised physical therapy program on a regular scheduled basis at least 3 times a week."** A list of durable medical equipment was similarly designed to maximize the amount that could be billed to insurance companies per patient. The Prognosis section was also preprinted; **it stated for each patient, regardless of actual condition, that the prognosis was "guarded,"**[13] that "the supporting tissues of the spine [would] become less effective," and that "chronic joint dysfunction" would likely ensue. In accordance with such directives, Keschner told his patients to return for treatment three or four times a week, thus maximizing no-fault insurance reimbursement.

Vinarsky programmed a computer to complete NF-3 No-Fault Insurance Law Verification of Treatment forms so as to indicate that the patient had not suffered from a similar

---

[12] Nowhere in any documents is it mentioned that any other chiropractor was charged in this case. Most likely it was a part-time doctor, who was not involved in any financial arrangements with Vinarsky, nor involved with any decision-making processes in the clinic, and simply saw patients that Keschner was also seeing. Nevertheless, even such limited involvement could become problematic and rise to the level of conspiracy, if it goes on long enough and an employee chiropractor could be expected to see that some patients and procedures were not legitimate.

[13] Boilerplate treatment plans are always a bad idea. Treatment plans should be tailored for each individual. At the very least, a pre-printed treatment plan form should have varied specific treatment options to choose from.

condition in the past and that the injury was the result of an automobile accident.

The NF-3 forms listed Keschner as the chiropractor, regardless of who had provided "treatment,"[14] and indicated that Goldman had provided biofeedback testing, range of motions tests, and physical therapy, even though these were in fact conducted by other staff, including one minimally trained billing employee.

II.

In November 2006, the police executed a search warrant at St. Nicholas Medical Clinic. Vinarsky kept the clinic open for about two weeks, but took no new patients. Around this time, Vinarsky opened a new clinic, sharing profits with Keschner again, in which Goldman had no part, but its existence was brief. Vinarsky closed both clinics, and there was no period of time in which either clinic continued to operate in his absence.

In February 2008, Keschner and Goldman were charged, in an 84-count indictment, with **enterprise corruption**, scheme to defraud in the first degree, and other crimes related to insurance fraud. Vinarsky was indicted as well. In 2009, after investigators executed search warrants at his apartment and at a law office, Vinarsky entered into a cooperation agreement. He pleaded guilty that December to enterprise corruption, grand larceny in the first degree, scheme to

---

[14] Block 16 of the NF-3 form requires the name and license number of the treating doctor if different than the billing provider. Misrepresentations in this field can meet the elements of Insurance Fraud- a false statement submitted to an insurer. This is obviously inconvenient when different chiropractors are treating patients every week, but that's not a good enough reason not to do it.

defraud in the first degree, and money laundering in the first degree.

The District Attorney's Office sent letters to the majority of the 54 former patients of St. Nicholas Medical Clinic whose names appeared in the indictment, informing them that the Office wished to speak with them about their visits to the clinic. Only three people indicated a willingness to speak with the People.

Keschner and Goldman proceeded to a joint jury trial, commencing in September 2010. A separate defense counsel represented each defendant. The prosecution theory was accomplice liability.

In his opening statement, the prosecutor explained that the jury would hear only from a "representative sample" of the patients treated at the clinic. He stated that the People had tried to contact "many" of "these patients . . . but they didn't want to talk to the District Attorney's Office, and you will understand why they didn't want to come and talk to the District Attorney's Office when it came time for us investigating this case." The jury subsequently heard testimony from a paralegal in the District Attorney's Office about her futile efforts to interview the patients.

Vinarsky's testimony spelled out the fraudulent scheme in detail. He insisted that he had never told Goldman or Keschner how to treat patients or what to prescribe, or discussed kickbacks or billing or other aspects of operations at the clinic with them. Vinarsky explained, however, that such conversations were unnecessary because, among other things, the **preprinted initial evaluation forms he created** told the doctors what treatment was "supposed to be done."[15]

As promised, the People also produced several witnesses who had been patients, with **legitimate**[16] or spurious injuries, at the clinic.

In addition to "chasing ambulances," **some of the runners employed by St. Nicholas Medical Clinic and their associates participated in staged car accidents.** One man who took part in such an accident, Hernandez, consulted at the clinic with a Dr. Hilaire, who diagnosed the uninjured man with numerous contusions and other trauma to his back and advised him to attend physical therapy three times a week, to use a thermophore, a lumbosacral orthosis, an orthopedic bed board, and an egg crate mattress, to have multiple X rays and MRIs, and to consult with a chiropractor, an acupuncturist, and an orthopedist. Hernandez saw Keschner a number of times; the chiropractor would either "crack" his back **or simply ask him how he was feeling and administer no treatment.**[17] NF-3 forms were submitted to GEICO on behalf of Hernandez for X rays, biofeedback training, chiropractic treatments, acupuncture sessions, and a cold water circulating unit. Eventually, Hernandez went to the authorities and admitted his involvement in the scheme.

---

[15] Never let a pre-printed form, or anyone else, dictate how a patient should be treated. If the form you are given is not adequate, hand-write your findings and plan, or design your own form.

[16] Of course there were patients with legitimate injuries, but that doesn't matter. It might have made Keschner feel like he was doing legitimate work, but it doesn't change the illegitimate nature of the larger situation.

[17] Since this occurred prior to the change to an RVU-based coding system, and the chiropractic code used for a visit was not specific, but simply a code for an "office visit" (99213), Keschner may have felt he was doing a reevaluation, and thus justified in billing for merely asking how a patient was feeling. Even if this were true, there should have been documentation to that effect sufficient to justify using that code.

A runner employed by St. Nicholas Medical Clinic named Perez testified that he had been "treated" at the clinic in connection with what the facility's medical records described as three separate motor vehicle accidents, in 2002, 2003 and 2004. In 2002, Goldman "evaluated" Perez and reported that he was suffering from post-concussion syndrome and a left shoulder injury; he wrote two prescriptions for durable medical equipment and advised Perez to get various tests, X rays and MRIs. Perez also received chiropractic "treatment" from Keschner. In 2003, Goldman "evaluated" Perez following another "accident"; he made the same report, without mentioning the 2002 incident, and wrote a prescription **for the same medical equipment**. Goldman also recommended chiropractic treatment four times a week, as well as X rays and MRIs, and referred Perez to an orthopedist, a neurologist, and a psychiatrist. In 2004, Goldman conducted the initial evaluation of Perez following a third "accident"; again **he used the same list of symptoms**, but added a knee injury. The same tests and equipment were prescribed as in previous years, as well as an additional MRI on Perez's knee. St. Nicholas Medical Clinic directly or indirectly billed rental car companies for all the expenses.

The jury heard testimony that another runner employed by St. Nicholas Medical Clinic became a paid confidential informant. He and two undercover officers went to the clinic with a fictitious accident report and documents suggesting insurance by GEICO. All three men saw Keschner, **who examined them cursorily and did not discuss diagnoses or treatment plans** for the invented minor pain symptoms they had reported. The next day, a physician at the clinic, Dr. Pone, recommended that the uninjured runner have a CT scan and an X ray, and prescribed an ankle brace, a cervical collar, and a special pillow. For several months, the men visited the clinic regularly, seeing a physical therapist and Keschner, who "cracked" their backs. The men were also given "biofeedback tests" but, as **video from a concealed**

camera revealed, only for a minute or two at a time and not in appropriate conditions. A neurologist who claimed to be administering electromyography **simply placed the needles on the undercovers' arms, without breaking the skin.**[18] When one of the undercovers told a receptionist at the clinic that he could not have an MRI she had recommended and suggested that he send his "brother" instead, the receptionist agreed. The same undercover, sent for an X ray, declined the procedure because the room he was directed to at the clinic was filthy and lacked standard protective equipment. The undercovers were periodically given pieces of durable medical equipment, including a special pillow, a heating pad, a lumbar support belt, a water cooler, an ankle brace, and an infrared heat lamp, but they were never told how to use the supplies. St. Nicholas Medical Clinic submitted NF-3s on behalf of the three men to GEICO, listing Goldman as the provider of the physical therapy and all tests, even though the men had never met Goldman.

In addition, the jury heard testimony from two, genuinely injured patients who were seen at St. Nicholas Medical Clinic.

One man, who had dislocated his kneecap, learned of the clinic through a lawyer. The clinic sent a driver to take the injured man to his first consultation. The physician, Pone, did not ask the patient how he had been injured, but recommended physical therapy three times a week, X rays and an MRI; receptionists at the clinic referred him to an acupuncturist and a physical therapist. **The patient also saw Keschner and another chiropractor, who administered "treatment" to his spine.** Eventually, the man's knee discomfort subsided. The clinic submitted NF-3s to MetLife

---

[18] This seems hard to believe, but nothing is impossible when it comes to fraud. Also, an undercover may have refused the needle portion to see if the doctor would "fake" the test so as not to lose the billing.

Insurance for treatment by St. Nicholas Medical Clinic, Keschner, and an acupuncturist.

A woman who had injured her arm when she was struck by a car was given the business card of an attorney, who recommended St. Nicholas Medical Clinic. The clinic sent a driver to pick her up. **Pone saw the patient, but did not examine her arm, and noted in medical records that she had sustained acute back trauma and a sprained shoulder and wrist.**[19] The woman was advised to attend physical therapy three times a week, have X rays and an MRI of her wrist, receive range of motion testing, use elbow and wrist support, and make appointments with an acupuncturist, an orthopedist, and a psychologist. During subsequent visits, the patient was instructed to take a number of pieces of durable medical equipment from a stack at the clinic, **but was not told how to use the supplies.**[20] Frustrated because of pressure to see specialists, including a psychologist, she stopped going to the clinic. The clinic submitted NF-3s to GMAC Insurance for both treatment and medical equipment, including a cold water circulating unit prescribed by Keschner.

A biostatistician who had reviewed 2,300 patient files recovered from the clinic testified that Goldman referred all of his patients to a neurologist and almost all to a chiropractor and a physical therapist. The expert also noted that Keschner prescribed four chiropractic visits per week to 93.3% of his patients, physical therapy to 94.4%,

---

[19] The doctor may have indeed examined the arm and wrist, but neglected to document it properly. And, as the axiom goes, "if it wasn't documented, it wasn't done." Always thoroughly document every area you examine, and if you don't examine it, document why not.

[20] If you prescribe or dispense DME (belts, collars, etc.), always instruct the patient in written form in the use of each item and keep a copy signed by the patient in the chart.

neurological or psychiatric consultation to 97.4%, MRIs to 97.5%, and X rays to 99.3%

The jury also heard expert testimony from a chiropractor that the treatment of the undercovers was not consistent with standard chiropractic care, would have accomplished no benefit, and may have been harmful if the men had actually been injured. Additionally, an expert testified that the number of tests ordered by clinic staff was greater than necessary, as was the quantity of medical equipment provided. **The expert disagreed with the "guarded" prognoses for patients whose medical conditions were improving**, and explained various respects in which entries in the clinic's medical records were, medically speaking, meaningless. All in all, the expert opined that many of the clinic's prognoses and prescriptions were inconsistent with the standard of care for physical medicine and rehabilitation.

A forensic accountant testified that the percentage of revenue from insurance companies paid to the clinic that was then transmitted by check to corporations controlled by Vinarsky was consistently 70%. **Keschner's corporations regularly paid 65% of money received to Vinarsky's corporations**.

At the close of the prosecution's case, Keschner's counsel moved to dismiss his enterprise corruption charge for lack of evidence that, absent Vinarsky's participation, the alleged enterprise could continue to exist. Supreme Court denied the motion, which Goldman's counsel did not join.

The defense then called character witnesses and one expert. Keschner and Goldman did not testify.

The jury found both defendants guilty of enterprise corruption, scheme to defraud in the first degree, grand larceny in the first degree (two counts), and money laundering in the second degree, **Keschner alone guilty of insurance fraud in the fourth degree (four counts) and**

falsifying business records in the first degree (two counts), and Goldman alone guilty of money laundering in the first degree, insurance fraud in the third degree (five counts), insurance fraud in the fourth degree (three counts), and falsifying business records in the first degree.

Keschner was probably a nice guy and a decent enough chiropractor. He may have thought that he was just doing what so many other chiropractors were doing—he had an opportunity to be in the no-fault business, and if that meant splitting profits with Vinarsky, well, that's the way the business worked. Patients came in with accident reports and told him they had pain; he took them at their word. Maybe he told himself that he didn't know how Vinarsky got patients, or that he didn't want to know, and it wasn't his job to know. Or, perhaps he just looked the other way. And certainly, there were legitimately injured patients, and they were probably nice people, and many of them no doubt liked Keschner and appreciated him.

In reality, while this all may have been true, Keschner's profit-splitting deal with Vinarsky gave him an interest in the operation, making him an accomplice to Vinarsky's crimes and implicating him in the "corrupt enterprise." His recordkeeping lapses and misrepresentations on insurance forms left him open to charges of Insurance Fraud and Falsifying Business Records.

Keschner was sentenced to one and a half to four years in state prison and $750,000 in fines. He appealed his conviction and lost. Goldman was sentenced to two and a half to seven and a half years and $800,000 in fines. Vinarsky, who had taken a plea deal to similar charges, was sentenced to three and a half to ten years in state prison.

No one thinks they're going to get caught. Many people don't even think they're doing anything wrong—or think that if they are, it's not a big deal, and everyone is doing it. In this case, the police were tipped off by one of the runners, who then became a confidential informant (CI). Keschner didn't have anything to do with the runners; he didn't hire them or pay them. It's likely he hardly even saw them, didn't know who they were, and never gave them much thought, but it was ultimately a runner that brought the operation down. The ensuing investigation took five years, using the CI and undercover detectives to gather evidence. Why did the runner decide to turn CI? We'll never know; maybe he regretted his participation in a life of crime. Or, maybe Vinarsky owed him money, and this was his way of getting revenge. It doesn't matter—what is important is not getting into a situation like this in the first place. If you follow the principles below, and the advice in the rest of this book, you will be able to practice no-fault with No Fear.

The "No Fear" Principles

- *Don't be a straw-owner, and don't enter a business association with those who use straw-owners. Know who you are working for and with, and use proper and legal terms in your business arrangements and associations.*

- *Don't perform unnecessary treatment, don't order unnecessary tests, and don't submit anything for billing that wasn't actually done or done properly.*

- *Document, document, document. Be meticulous in your charting.*

- *Don't overtreat patients. Don't let anyone dictate how or how often you treat patients. Don't see patients whom you suspect are not legitimately injured, and if you're working in a clinic where you suspect that many patients are not, you're probably working in the wrong clinic.*

- *Never allow yourself to be put in a position where you cannot give a good answer to the question of why you did or did not do something with a patient; always ask yourself what your treatment rationale is, as if you were being cross-examined.*

- *Treat patients the way you would want a family member to be treated—objectively, and with clinical goals foremost in mind rather than pecuniary interests or satisfying quotas, and everything else will take care of itself.*

III

IN THE CLINIC

"I have never considered it beneath my dignity to do anything to relieve human suffering."
—Daniel David Palmer, Founder of Chiropractic

7

EXCELLENCE IN THE CLINIC

As a chiropractor, you were trained to heal. You studied the entire human organism, from the biochemistry of the smallest cellular organelle to all the muscles, bones, and organs. You traced every nerve throughout the body, committing its map to memory. You pored through the myriad afflictions a person could have. You learned how to take and read x-rays, examining them for the minutest details and listening for the secrets the body would whisper to you through them. You were taught the relationship of the spine and nervous system to health and disease, and how to analyze and adjust the spine to influence healing in the body. You delved into the intricacies of nutrition and wellness. You worked and you studied and you learned. You envisioned helping families and their children optimize their health through the distinct science and art of chiropractic.

And now you're in the south Bronx for ten hours a day, seeing people who've been rear-ended in car accidents.

I know; I've been there. So, if you'll pardon the cliché, I feel your pain. But the fact is, while at times you may not be able to help feeling like a cog in a machine, chiropractors fill an important role in the treatment of accident injuries that no other practitioner does. That is, if we do our job properly.

As health professionals, chiropractors are unique; we lay hands on a patient more and longer than most others. We see them frequently, and we get up close to them, talk to them, and get to know them. Practicing chiropractic in a personal injury clinic is an opportunity to bring chiropractic care to hundreds, or thousands, of patients a year who may have never had it and otherwise likely never would. Personally, I have found no-fault work to be rewarding—many patients respond beautifully to adjustments, and it is gratifying to see a patient's face light up after an adjustment and get up from the table saying how much better they feel. Sometimes we catch something seriously wrong with a patient that is beyond our abilities and are able to get them the help they need. Not everyone is out to scam the system; many people are genuinely hurt in car accidents, and this is the time in their lives when they need us to be the best at what we do.

I won't tell you it hasn't ever been frustrating, or depressing, or even demoralizing; I can recall many days working in an 8x10 foot windowless room for ten hours a day, with a torn vinyl bench and a detached 16" roll of paper, as upwards of 60 patients trooped through. Some of them barely spoke English, and some of them barely spoke at all. But even in places like that, there were bright moments, like when a patient who had never been "osseously" adjusted before would get up after an adjustment and say, "Wow!" Those are the moments that matter.

Clinical excellence is the cornerstone of what we do; it is, to use another somewhat cliched expression, "where the rubber meets the road." Its title notwithstanding, the previous section of this book may have scared you a little. That's OK—

that's what it was intended to do. But this section will focus on the patient, and on the application of the science and art of chiropractic to achieve clinical excellence in treating automobile accident injuries.

Automobile Accident Injuries

The kind of injuries that you will typically see in a no-fault practice will run the gamut from mild, inconveniencing soft tissue injuries all the way to fractures, torn knees and shoulders, and more. (You won't necessarily be treating some of those injuries, but the patients you will be adjusting will have them.) Some patients will deal with more severe injuries well, and some patients with minor complaints will find them highly bothersome. It may be tempting to view a patient who was in a seemingly minor "fender-bender" with no major injuries as not being significantly hurt. But even seemingly mundane accidents that don't cause major vehicle damage can cause serious injuries that take months to heal.[21]

Counterintuitively, even collisions with a delta V of as low as 6-9 mph can cause painful and significant injuries.[22] Very low-level accelerations can cause cervical and lumbar disc herniations, and there is no established minimum threshold for significant injury.[23] It's important to keep this in mind

---

[21] Croft, Arthur C., and Michael D. Freeman. Correlating crash severity with injury risk, injury severity, and long-term symptoms in low velocity motor vehicle collisions. Medical Science Monitor 11.10 (2005): RA316-RA321.

[22] Croft, A. C. The biomechanical and kinematic differences between rear impact and frontal impact automobile crashes at low velocities. Journal of Biomechanics 39 (2006): S145.

[23] Freeman, Michael D., et al. Significant spinal injury resulting from low-level accelerations: a case series of roller coaster injuries. Archives of Physical Medicine and Rehabilitation 86.11 (2005): 2126-2130.

when practicing in an accident clinic, since considering the industry's reputation, one may be inclined to think that just because a patient is not incapacitated with pain, or does not have obvious disfigurement, it means that they are not significantly injured.

Patients presenting to a chiropractor after a motor vehicle accident will most commonly complain of pain in the neck, thoracolumbar spine, or both. Some may also report headaches, which may be cervical in origin. The neck and back symptoms may or may not radiate to an extremity, and may or may not also produce paresthesia (numbness and tingling) in an extremity. A careful and thorough interview and initial examination are essential; asking the right questions and employing the right examination techniques will allow you to more accurately plan and document the patient's course of chiropractic treatment.

8

PATIENT INTAKE

Forms

All patients complete a chiropractic intake form when they first arrive at the clinic. The formats vary, but aside from general demographic information, all forms typically ask for information such as:

- Date of accident
- If the patient was a driver, passenger, or pedestrian, and location in the vehicle (if a passenger)
- Seat belt use
- Direction/location of impact
- Loss of consciousness and airbag deployment
- Prehospital care, hospital transport

Patients will sometimes have completed this form prior to seeing you, but sometimes will have not, and will complete it with you at the initial visit. Make sure all questions are answered completely.

No-Fault Assignment

Some clinics will have this done before the patient sees you, but in some clinics, the patient will be given the form by the DC at the initial visit. The NF-AOB, as we mentioned earlier, assigns the patient's benefits to the provider or provider's P.C. for direct reimbursement. It also assigns the rights to contest claim denials and litigate denied claims for treatment.

HIPAA

The Health Insurance Portability and Accountability Act of 1996 sets forth the rules and procedures surrounding the protection and transmission of protected health information (PHI). No fault clinics are not exempt from them. If your practice, or the practice you are employed by, transmits PHI electronically (which includes email or fax, it is considered a "covered entity" subject to the Privacy Rule. Patients also have certain rights under the law and must be informed of them. The clinic should have all its Privacy Policies readily available for review, and ideally, you as a chiropractor (or your chiropractor employer) should as well. Patients should receive a Notice of Privacy Practices and sign an acknowledgment that he or she has received it, as well as an authorization to release information for outside treatment, payment, and operations. A comprehensive listing of HIPAA resources and documents can be found at:

https://www.hhs.gov/hipaa/forprofessionals/index.html.

Informed Consent

This is something that seems to be sorely missing among chiropractors in many no-fault clinics. Aside from being required, it's also a good idea. Adverse effects of adjustments can and do happen, and many patients in a no-fault clinic have already demonstrated a willingness to be litigious. A simple informed consent form goes a long way toward protecting you. A sample informed consent form can be found in Appendix B of this book.

Minor Consent

Children under the age of 18 get into accidents too. Usually, they come in to the office for the first time with their parents, but not always, especially in some areas. Also, they may have come with their parents on their first visit to the clinic when they saw the MD, but by the time they see you, they are there on their own.

Never see a child, even for an initial examination, without a signed consent form in the chiropractic file. The minor consent should be specific to chiropractic and to the clinic you are in. The best practice is to have the minor consent on the same page as the chiropractic informed consent form. A sample minor consent form can be found in Appendix B of this book.

> *I had just begun a part-time job working for another chiropractor in two different offices. In one, he had just "taken over the P.C." for another chiropractor who had just left, and apparently, taken all of his patient records with him. (This is usually a bad sign—see chapter 16.) This meant that every patient had to be examined as a new patient, even though some of them*

had been coming to this facility for months. It was laborious work, and the patients, who were not told anything about the change, were understandably annoyed about it too. Sometimes, I would have access to a patient's medical chart so at least I would be able to see some of their histories. But mostly, they would just wander into my room after their therapy, looking confused. One young man wandered in, and as I had him complete paperwork it became apparent that he was only sixteen years old. I stopped the proceedings and informed him and the management that I would be unable to see him until there was a signed informed consent for chiropractic treatment.

When I spoke to my absentee employer, later on, I told him that we would need to have minor consent forms (and while we were at it, a general chiropractic treatment consent form—there was none in the paperwork he supplied me). His response was, "Oh, yeah, yeah." I made my own combined form (see Appendix B) and brought it to both offices, and he never supplied me with one.

I only stayed with that employer for a few more weeks, finally quitting after he messed up the very first payroll (see chapter 16).

Pain Diagram

A pain diagram is a wonderful tool that too many clinics and chiropractors aren't using. It provides a visual representation, in the patient's own rendering, of the nature and location of their symptoms. Aside from the obvious reasons for using one, it can also be referred to as a baseline if the patient later complains of or mentions a symptom that wasn't reported initially, but he or she claims was. It can also be used at regular intervals during the course of treatment as a progress and outcomes assessment tool. Aside from the "stick figure" human outline form for marking the location of symptoms, the pain diagram should have a visual analog pain scale for recording severity. This is a line along which patients mark the severity of pain, from "no pain" on the left to "unbearable pain" on the right. Unlike a numerical 1-10 pain scale, which patients can exaggerate, there are no numbers—just a straight line. These measurements can again be observed over time as a progress assessment tool. The patient should sign and date the form, and the chiropractor should initial it and keep it in the file.

NO-FAULT WITH NO FEAR

9

INITIAL INTERVIEW & HISTORY

The initial interview establishes the basic circumstances of the accident, such as the direction and velocity of impact, any hospital care, and the symptoms he or she is experiencing. It also will reveal other important details such as past or current other medical history, including previous accidents, injuries, or surgeries. All of these will direct the particular chiropractic approach you will take towards treatment.

In many clinics, patients will see the medical doctor before they see the chiropractor. Sometimes they will see both on the same visit, but it is better if the visits are on separate days, so as not to overwhelm the patient. Bills for evaluation services are also less likely to be questioned when Evaluation and Management (E&M) services are done on separate visits. If possible, review the medical doctor's initial report or notes before or while you are interviewing the new patient; it will help guide your interview and examination.

Very often, new patients will enter the clinic who do not speak English as their native language—usually, it will be Spanish but can be any other language. There will sometimes be a relative with the patient or a clinic staff member who can translate for them during the interview and examination. Do not interview or examine a new patient with whom you cannot adequately communicate. If no one is available to translate, defer seeing that patient until such time as a translator becomes available—it may have to be at another visit. If there is a translator, indicate in the chart that the interview was conducted with a translator, and who that translator was (staff member, relative, etc.).

Basic Accident Information

After you greet the patient and introduce yourself, review with the patient, from the intake form, the basic circumstances of the accident: was the patient a pedestrian, driver or passenger, if a passenger where they were seated in the vehicle, direction of impact, loss of consciousness, seat belt use, hospital transport, etc. Ask about any tests or imaging studies done at the hospital, and any medications prescribed. Inquire if the patient has had treatment anywhere else prior to coming to your clinic. Also, it is a good idea to ask if the accident occurred during the course of the patient's employment—if it did, it would be considered a Worker's Compensation case, which would not be reimbursable under no-fault.

Chief Complaints

Ask the patient where they are having pain. Use the pain diagram to direct your questioning, comparing their answers with their diagram markings, and clarify any discrepancies or ambiguities. Use the patient's own words, in quotes, when writing your initial report.

Ask if their pain travels anywhere. Don't ask leading questions, such as: "Does the pain go down your arm?" or, "Do you have pain in your lower back?" Some patients may magnify symptoms or be led to answer positively when they don't really have a complaint. If the patient tells you that they have pain in their neck, shoulder, and arm, it may require further questioning to tease out whether the pain is cervical in origin with radiation to the shoulder and arm, or separate neck, shoulder and arm complaints.

If the patient complains of a headache, ask and note the location, character, frequency, and intensity of the pain. Patients will also frequently complain of non-spinal areas of pain after an auto accident, most commonly knee, shoulder, and wrist pain. Note these areas of pain, but since as a chiropractor you will not be treating non-spinal areas, you need not examine them; just note that examination of those areas was deferred to the appropriate specialist. (I often examine the shoulder anyway, to differentiate between lower neck pain with referral to the shoulder, or trapezius strain, and a rotator cuff injury; see the section on examination techniques.)

Past Medical and Health History

This is a crucial part of the initial interview that is important not to skim over. Ask about any current or past medical problems, and give examples: i.e., "diabetes, high blood pressure, thyroid problems?" Ask what medications they are taking, including over-the-counter medications and contraceptives, and any vitamin supplements. Inquire if there are any medications they should be taking, but are not; patients commonly go off their hypertension meds and psychiatric meds. Patients on anticoagulants are at elevated risk for bruising and bleeding, and you should probably not adjust their cervical spine manually.

Inquire about current or past use of alcohol, drugs, and smoking. Some patients may not be entirely candid, but some will. Smokers have a higher risk of developing lower back pain[24] and have a higher risk for their pain becoming chronic.[25]

Question the patient about any surgical history. For some reason, some patients only answer about any abdominopelvic or thoracic surgery (to them, this is what "surgery" means)—so ask specifically about any broken bones, gunshot wounds, etc. A good question to ask is, "have you ever been admitted to the hospital for any reason?"

> *Patients can be funny about what they tell you and don't tell you about their histories. It's not necessarily that they want to hide it-—although there are patients who do. It's just that for some reason, they forget to tell you things, or it doesn't register that something could be significant. For example, I once was interviewing an older woman in her 60s. I asked her the typical questions but probably neglected to specifically ask about broken bones. She mentioned some minor surgical procedures, and we moved on to the examination. During the exam, she offhandedly made a comment about her "bad leg." I asked her what she meant, and she replied that she had had a*

---

[24] Goldberg, M. S., Scott, S. C., & Mayo, N. E. (2000). A review of the association between cigarette smoking and the development of nonspecific back pain and related outcomes. Spine, 25(8), 995-1014.

[25] Petre, B., Torbey, S., Griffith, J. W., De Oliveira, G., Herrmann, K., Mansour, A., & Apkarian, A. V. (2015). Smoking increases risk of pain chronification through shared corticostriatal circuitry. Human brain mapping, 36(2), 683-694.

motorcycle accident many decades ago as a young woman in India, and she had fractured her tibia in several places, requiring a metal rod to be inserted. In checking the MD's notes, I saw that this had not been mentioned anywhere—she hadn't told him either. Furthermore, he had ordered MRIs for her. I left a note for the MD to consider changing the orders to a CT scan, and I also let the patient know that she should probably not have an MRI. I also made a note for myself that any leg length analysis would probably be unreliable on this patient.

Another time (much earlier in practice), I saw a young man who categorically denied any past medical or surgical history. I took him for x-rays, and as I put them up on the box, I saw a bullet lodged near his spine.

Ask about any prior automobile accidents, if there were any injuries, and if there are any residual symptoms from any other accidents. For many, this will not be their first accident.

A question I always find useful to ask is, "have you ever seen a chiropractor before?" Many never have. Some may, especially if they've had a prior car accident and have already been through this before in another clinic. If they have, ask what kind of techniques the chiropractor may have used—it may surprise you to hear that they were never adjusted manually.

I was interviewing a patient who had told me that he had a previous accident a couple of years prior, but that he had sustained no injuries except for his right knee. He had denied any past surgical history except for an arthroscopic procedure on that knee related to that accident. So far, so good.

I then asked him if he had ever seen a chiropractor before, and he said that he had. I asked what for, and he replied, "after that accident."

When I asked why he had seen a chiropractor after an accident where he had denied injuring anything but his knee, he stammered and said he didn't know why.

It's impossible to say for sure, but instances like this may be an indication that there was some less than honest activity in the past. Or the present. Or, he could have simply misinterpreted what I meant by "injury." In any event, it's important to conduct a thorough interview to get the most complete picture possible of a patient's current problem and past history. Incongruent answers to questions, like these, should make your examination more deliberate, and you more wary of incongruent examination findings that suggest nonorganic complaints.

10

EXAMINATION

Components of the Examination

Observation

The examination begins with observation. Note the patient's general appearance, level of alertness, and apparent degree of distress. Take note of the patient's body language while they are in the waiting area. Study their gait as they walk into the exam room. Is it stiff and guarded? Do they appear to have limited range of motion? If they drop something, can they pick it up easily or are they slow and stiff? Watch for an antalgic gait or lean, and Trendelenburg, steppage, shuffling, or wide-based or other neurological gait. Correlate your observations with your examination findings later.

Vital Signs

Record the patient's height and weight. Take the patient's pulse (heart) rate, respiratory rate, and blood pressure, and record your findings. If the BP is high, as it often is, check it several times over the next few visits to rule out "white coat hypertension." If it stays high, advise the patient to see his or her primary physician, and make a written note that you have done so. Patients are often unaware that they have elevated blood pressure because it has almost no symptoms, so they don't check it. (On several occasions I have seen new patients with headaches and high blood pressure sent to the ER by ambulance, to be safe.) Chiropractors can be the ones to alert the patient to this and ensure that the appropriate referral is made. A simple and inexpensive digital blood pressure machine can take both pressure and heart rate measurements.

Palpation

Palpate the patient's areas of complaint. This is the first laying on of hands; feel for muscle spasm and hypertonicity and ask about tenderness. If it's part of your technique, you can use motion palpation, testing joint play. Feel the paraspinal muscles, spinous processes, and other surrounding musculature and tissues. Note your findings. Tenderness can be graded numerically I-IV, or as mild, moderate, or severe. A chiropractic palpatory examination can also be incorporated here.

Range of Motion (ROM)

Assess the patient's active and passive ROM for each area of complaint in all planes and rotation. I usually have the patient stand first, and check lumbar ROM by having the patient bend slowly at the waist toward their toes, as far as possible, even with some pain. This is repeated in all other planes and rotation. Next assess cervical ROM, first asking them to perform active ROM in all planes, and then placing your hands on their head and passively rotating it gently throughout all ranges of motion. Note your findings; ROM can be assessed with use of a goniometer, but many doctors simply observe the ROM and estimate the degree of movement. If you do this, make a note that all ranges of motion were obtained via observation. Also, note if pain was reported throughout the ROM or only at end range. I have seen many different references for "normal" ROM, but the most important reference is what is normal for that patient; a short endomorphic individual with "no neck" is not going to have the same range of motion as a lanky ectomorph.

Cervical ROM can be tested while standing behind the seated patient, and from there it is easy to move directly to cervical orthopedic testing.

Orthopedic Testing

While it's beyond the scope of this book to provide an exhaustive catalog of every orthopedic test, there are those that are routinely used and that commonly appear on clinic exam forms.

Cervical Distraction—a useful test that can also be therapeutic. Standing behind the patient, cup the head in both hands with your thumbs under the patient's mastoid processes and your fingers in front of their ears. This avoids cupping under the jaw or neck, which patients may find awkward or uncomfortable. Exert gentle traction upward (+y axis) for at least 10 seconds. If traction relieves pain, there is most likely a foraminal encroachment, joint capsule irritation, and/or disc involvement. Pain returning once traction is stopped confirms this. If the traction produces pain, that indicates muscle and soft tissue involvement. Note your findings—but simply indicating "positive" or "negative' for this test does not provide any useful information; indicate what reaction the test produced.[26] Example: "Cervical distraction resulted in reduction of patient's radiating right arm pain."

Cervical Compression—part of a standard cervical assessment, this test is particularly useful when there are arm symptoms along with neck pain. It should not be performed when there has been direct trauma or with rheumatoid arthritis, or when cervical instability or fracture is suspected. Standing behind the patient, place your hands on top of the head and exert gentle, yet increasing downward pressure (-y axis). This will usually aggravate reported neck and/or arm symptoms. The compression can be combined with lateral flexion and extension, rotation to the symptomatic side (Jackson's compression), or rotation, lateral flexion and extension (maximum foraminal compression). Induction or reproduction of arm pain, numbness or paresthesia is strongly indicative of radiculopathy, with a herniated disc being the likely cause (especially in patients under 60). Local pain only suggests disc derangement, facet syndrome, or segmental dysfunction (chiropractic subluxation).

As before, proper documentation goes beyond simply indicating a "positive" or "negative" test—document the results, describing the neck position, symptoms produced, which side was affected, and the pattern of pain radiation.[27] Example: "Maximum foraminal compression on the right produced sharp pain radiating to the right thumb and forefinger."

---

[26] Hoppenfeld S. Physical Examination of the Spine and Extremities. San Mateo, CA: Appleton & Lange, 1976.

[27] Magee DJ. Orthopedic Physical Assessment, 3rd ed. Philadelphia, PA: WB Saunders; 1997.

(Note that a report of low back pain in response to cervical compression is one of Waddell's signs,[28] and is considered a sign of non-organic, or psychological etiology of pain—or, alternatively, a "behavioral response or reaction to a physical examination."[29] It is one of five signs, and three positive signs is considered significant. Waddell's signs are controversial,[30] and positive findings do not exclude organic pathology, but three or more positive signs have a positive correlation with depression, hysteria, and symptom magnification.[31])

Shoulder Depression—this is a test for nerve root or brachial plexus impingement in patients who have neck and radiating upper extremity symptoms. It's a very commonly listed test on clinic examination forms, even though Bakody's is better for that purpose.

With the patient seated or supine, ask the patient to bend their head toward the side opposite their arm symptoms as far as possible. Stabilize the head with one hand, and with the other, depress the affected shoulder. Radicular pain on the depressed side is a positive test. Confirm by relaxing the pressure on the shoulder until the radicular symptoms subside, then have the patient rotate their head away from the depressed shoulder. Return of the radicular symptoms is

---

[28] Waddell, Gordon; John McCulloch; Ed Kummel; Robert Venner (March–April 1980). "Nonorganic Physical Signs in Low-Back Pain." Spine. 5 (2): 117–125.

[29] Main, Chris; Gordon Waddell (November 1998). "Behavioral Responses to Examination: A Reappraisal of the Interpretation of 'Nonorganic Signs'." Spine. 23 (21): 2367–2371.

[30] Fishbain, David; R. B. Cutler; H. L. Rosomoff; R. Steele Rosomoff (November–December 2004). "Is There a Relationship Between Nonorganic Physical Findings (Waddell Signs) and Secondary Gain/Malingering?"

[31] Maruta T, Goldman S, Chan CW, Ilstrup DM, Kunselman AR, Colligan RC. (1997). "Waddell's nonorganic signs and Minnesota Multiphasic Personality Inventory profiles in patients with chronic low back pain." Spine. 22 (1): 72–5.

confirmation. Again, note your findings descriptively; local pain should also be notated.

Soto-Hall—is a nonspecific test of the lower cervical and upper thoracic spine when there is a suspected fracture or other injury. With the patient supine, place pressure on the sternum to keep the torso neutral and flex the patient's head toward the chest. Local pain suggests bone or joint injury, and may also cause pain from muscular or ligamentous injury. Watch for meningeal tension signs such as Lhermitte's and Lindner's (pain shooting down the spine or lower extremities). Again, record specific results. Example: "Soto-Hall testing elicited sharp local cervicothoracic pain with no lower extremity reaction."

Kemp's Test—Kemp's is commonly listed on almost every clinic's initial examination form. It is also known as the "facet loading test" and is a provocative maneuver that loads the lumbar spinal facet joints. It can be performed with the patient standing or seated. Place your hand on the patient's iliac crest opposite the side being tested. With your hand on the patient's shoulder on the side being tested, bend the patient's torso into ipsilateral extension, rotation, and lateral flexion and hold for at least three seconds, noting any report and location of pain.

This is a highly nonspecific test,[32] and is also not considered to be very accurate in localizing the specific pain generating tissue or structure.[33] In my opinion, this test simply confirms that a patient has back pain—it's not diagnostic of anything. I have never seen a patient in a no-fault clinic with low back pain who didn't also have a positive

---

[32] Craig E. Morris; Low back syndromes; McGraw-hill professional; 2005

[33] Stuber K, Lerede C, Kristmanson K, Sajko S, Bruno P. The diagnostic accuracy of the Kemp's test: a systematic review. J Can Chiropr Assoc. 2014 Sep; 58(3): 258–267.

Kemp's test. Which is probably why lawyers like seeing it on a clinic exam form—it will always be positive.

Straight Leg Raise (SLR)—this is also known as Lasegue's test. The SLR test is done to establish or rule out a radiculopathy caused by a herniated lumbar disc in a patient with low back pain and is highly sensitive for those indications.[34]

This is important; not all patients with lower back pain have a herniated lumbar disc, and not all patients with a herniated lumbar disc will have lower back pain or radicular leg pain. *A positive test is only radiating lower extremity pain (usually sciatic pain), extending below the knee, between 30 and 70 degrees of leg raising.* That's it. Low back pain only, tight hamstrings, or hip or groin pain, while they should be noted, do not constitute a positive SLR. I have seen many charts that have a positive SLR noted when the patient has low back pain only. It is also important to note that while a highly *sensitive* test, it does not have very high *specificity* for diagnosing herniated discs.[35]

With the patient supine, slowly raise the patient's leg. I always ask them to "let me know if you have pain anywhere." If they wince or report pain, stop the leg raise and ask where. Note the degree of leg raise where the pain was reported. Again, record a positive straight leg raise only if the patient reports sharp radiating lower extremity pain below the knee between 30 and 70 degrees of leg raise. If the patient reports only lower back pain, buttock pain, hip pain, or "pulling" behind the leg, record the results as well. Example: "Negative straight leg raising on the right, with local low back and right buttock pain reported at 45 degrees." Or:

---

[34] Devillé WL, van der Windt DA, Dzaferagić A, Bezemer PD, Bouter LM. The test of Lasègue: systematic review of the accuracy in diagnosing herniated discs.Spine. 2000; 25:1140-7.

[35] *Supra*, Note 34.

Ø R SLR w/ loc LBP & R buttock pain @ 45°

If the SLR is positive, confirm with **Braggard's** test. Lower the leg approximately 10 degrees below the reported level of pain and dorsiflex the ankle. You can also have the patient flex their neck toward their chest. Both increase meningeal tension and will increase radicular pain due to impingement at the spinal dorsal nerve root, and confirm the SLR.

You can also perform the seated leg raise. With the patient seated on the table, extend the patient's lower leg at the knee toward full extension. If there is a dorsal nerve root impingement the patient will report shooting radicular pain from the lower back below the knee and may lean backward to reduce dural tension on the nerve. The seated SLR is also known as one of Waddell's signs,[36] and he suggests performing the seated SLR to detect possible behavioral responses to examination. This can be done by letting the patient know you will be examining their knee, or when you perform deep tendon reflexes at the knee, and then casually do a seated SLR. It can also be used to confirm a positive supine SLR, but as a standalone test for radiculopathy, it is not as sensitive as the classic supine straight leg raise.[37]

A variation on the seated leg raise is **Bechterew's test**— here the patient actively extends their own knees fully, one side at a time, and then both together. This may produce radicular pain in the case of a disc herniation with dorsal root impingement. It can also produce lower back pain. Findings should be recorded descriptively and specifically.

---

[36] *Supra,* Note 28.

[37] Rabin A, Gerszten PC, Karausky P, et al. The sensitivity of the seated straight-leg raise test compared with the supine straight-leg raise test in patients presenting with magnetic resonance imaging evidence of lumbar nerve root compression. Arch Phys Med Rehabil, 2007;88(7):840-3.

In terms of exam flow, many procedures can be done without requiring much or any change in either examiner or patient position—for example, the seated leg raise, Bechterew's test, knee and ankle deep tendon reflexes, and manual motor strength testing of the lower extremity can all be rapidly done in a short time with almost no change in position.

Not every possible test needs to be done with every patient; it's not necessary to perform several tests for radiculopathy if there's a conclusive result after one or two. If a patient has a negative straight leg raise, there's no need to perform a Braggard's test.

Other Tests—there are many other orthopedic tests that can be employed during an examination to assess the spine and extremities: Hibb's and Ely's tests (for sacroiliac pain), Apley's and Yergason's tests (for shoulder pain), McMurray's test (for knee pain). However, these are the most commonly used tests in assessing the chiropractic patient following an automobile accident. Since chiropractors in New York generally do not treat injuries to extremities, and since all no-fault clinics have a physical therapist and a medical doctor, I personally do not usually examine or perform extremity orthopedic tests (sometimes I will test the shoulder to differentiate it from a neck complaint). In the case of extremity complaints, note the complaint and indicate that examination and treatment of the extremity is deferred to the MD and PT.

Neurologic Assessment

Evaluate the patient's neurological status, beginning with the cranial nerves. In straightforward cases, this can often be done largely via simple observation of the patient's face; look for symmetry of facial expression, smooth and symmetrical eye movements, and be aware of any speech deficits and any indication that the patient has trouble hearing. That will mostly cover CN III through XII, and any gaps can be filled in as you conduct the rest of the examination. Cranial nerve deficits after an auto accident are not a very common presentation in no-fault clinics. In your notes, you can indicate that CN III-XII appeared normal on gross observation. Of course, if you suspect a cranial nerve lesion or if other complaints or findings warrant it, you should conduct a more detailed cranial nerve assessment.

Neurologic testing will include deep tendon reflexes at the patellar, Achilles, brachioradialis, biceps, and triceps tendons bilaterally. Responses are graded as follows:

0 = no response; always abnormal
1+ = slight but visible response; may or may not be normal
2+ = brisk response; normal
3+ = very brisk response; may or may not be normal
4+ = tap elicits a repeating reflex (clonus); always abnormal

Responses of 0 and 1+ are hyporeflexia, which usually suggests a lesion or injury involving one or more parts of the two-neuron spinal reflex arc. Responses of 3+ and 4+ are hyperreflexia, which can indicate a lesion in corticospinal and other descending spinal pathways, above the level of the reflex pathway (also called an upper motor neuron lesion).

Reflex responses can sometimes be difficult to elicit, especially in anxious patients. Vary your position and the position of the limb to be tested. The patient can also employ the Jendrassik maneuver to bring out the reflex response. Asymmetrically diminished reflex responses (side to side differences) are more concerning than symmetrically diminished responses.[38]

---

[38] Walker HK. Deep Tendon Reflexes. In: Walker HK, Hall WD, Hurst JW, editors. Clinical Methods: The History, Physical, and Laboratory Examinations. 3rd edition. Boston: Butterworths; 1990. Chapter 72.

Patients who are on certain antidepressant and other psychotropic medications can exhibit abnormal reflexes, and this can be an indication of a condition known as serotonin syndrome, which can be life-threatening.[39] (I once saw a patient who was on several antidepressant medications exhibit repeated ankle clonus, and after conferring with her personal physician, he told me that it was most likely an adverse effect of long-term use of the medication.) Antidepressant use is very prevalent in the general population,[40] so it's not far-fetched that you might see a patient with an abnormal reflex response and be in a position to actually save a life. All the more reason to take a detailed and thorough history, including all current medications.

Occasionally, you will not be able to assess certain deep tendon reflexes—the patient may have a knee or ankle injury or swelling or be in a splint or other restrictive device. Record that the specific reflex was not tested and why.

Sensory Examination

The sensory examination is part of a complete assessment of patients complaining of neck or back pain with extremity symptoms. Some patients will complain of pain radiating from the neck or lower back into their arm or leg, and will also complain of numbness and/or tingling sensations. *Numbness* means diminished sensation, and *tingling* is a pins-and-needles feeling, which is also called *paresthesia*. Patients sometimes confuse the two, and it is helpful to explain the difference to them when asking about those symptoms.

---

[39] Frank C. Recognition and treatment of serotonin syndrome. Canadian Family Physician. 2008;54(7):988-992.

[40] Pratt LA, Brody DJ, Gu Q. Antidepressant Use in Persons Aged 12 and Over: United States, 2011–2014. NCHS (CDC) Data Brief No.283, August 2017.

I have found that very often, pain radiation will not be described along "textbook" dermatome patterns. Patients will frequently describe pain radiating down an extremity differently, and will also commonly report symptoms like diffuse numbness and/or tingling in an entire hand or foot, or sometimes a location like the upper thigh. I have even had patients report numbness in their back. These patterns of sensory disturbance are not classically dermatomal, and may not necessarily be radicular. There is also some dermatomal overlap and variability; classical dermatome maps do not always correspond to actual skin surface sensory representations.[41]

In the clinic, what you will probably find is that most often, at the initial examination patients will report sensory disturbance rather than sensory loss. Unless there is a severe nerve compression (which you will suspect from the history and the rest of the presentation), patients coming into the clinic within a short time of an accident will not yet have had time to develop profound sensory loss. This makes it even more important to conduct follow up examinations at regular intervals to monitor progression of symptoms, in case it manifests later on.

Sensation can be tested on the upper and lower extremities with a pinwheel, or even an unbent paperclip, using the bent side for dull and the exposed end for sharp sensation. There is some variability, but the general dermatome locations for the upper extremity are: C5—upper lateral arm; C6—lateral forearm and first two fingers; C7—middle finger and the center of the palm; C8—lower medial forearm and 5th finger; T1—upper medial forearm; and T2, upper medial arm. In the lower extremity: L3—anterior thigh

---

[41] Slipman CW, Plastaras CT, Palmitier RA, et al. Symptom provocation of fluoroscopically guided cervical nerve root stimulation. Are dynatomal maps identical to dermatomal maps? Spine, 1998;23(20):2235-42.

above the knee; L4—leg medial to the tibia and medial big toe; L5—lower leg lateral to the tibia and dorsum of the foot; S1, lateral foot and 5th toe. Use the sharper and dull edges of the paperclip on both extremities and ask the patient if they are feeling the appropriate sensation, and if it feels very different side to side. Don't be surprised if you get some unsure or hesitant responses. However, if the patient is uncertain if there is a difference, there probably isn't any. Record your findings in the chart.

Occasionally, as with reflexes, you will not be able to test certain dermatomes—patients may have other injuries, and may be in a cast or sling, have bandages, abrasions, or skin lesions that preclude dermatome testing. Note in the chart that the area was not tested for sensation, along with the reason.

Motor Testing

The motor examination in the context of the no-fault clinic is mainly to assess for the presence of motor deficit caused by radiculopathy. Keep in mind, however, that as with sensory deficits, most patients will be presenting to the clinic too early to be experiencing profound motor deficits. Again, unless their history and presentation raise your suspicion, you should probably not expect to see motor deficit at the initial examination in most cases. And, as with sensory testing, follow up motor examinations at regular intervals is vital to catch any deficit if it does develop later on, especially if the patient is not progressing satisfactorily.

Manual motor testing responses are graded using a 0-5 strength scale (see Table 1) as follows:

Grade 0: No movement.
Grade 1: Trace of contraction, but no movement at the joint.
Grade 2: Movement at the joint with gravity eliminated.
Grade 3: Movement against gravity, but not resistance.
Grade 4: Movement against resistance, but with less strength.
Grade 5: Full strength against resistance.

Table 1: Manual Muscle Grading

Key to Muscle Grading

	Function of the Muscle		Grade	
No Movement	No contractions felt in the muscle	0	0	Zero
	Tendon becomes prominent or feeble contraction felt in the muscle, but no visible movement of the part	T	1	Trace
Test Movement	**MOVEMENT IN HORIZONTAL PLANE**			
	Moves through partial range of motion	1	2-	Poor-
	Moves through complete range of motion	2	2	Poor
Test Position	**ANTIGRAVITY POSITION**			
	Moves through partial range of motion	3	2+	
	Gradual release from test position	4	3-	Fair-
	Holds test position (no added pressure)	5	3	Fair
	Holds test position against slight pressure	6	3+	Fair+
	Holds test position against slight to moderate pressure	7	4-	Good-
	Holds test position against moderate pressure	8	4	Good
	Holds test position against moderate to strong pressure	9	4+	Good+
	Holds test position against strong pressure	10	5	Normal

Modified from 1993 Florence P. Kendall. Author grants permission to reproduce this chart

To assess motor weakness due to compromise of specific spinal nerve roots, a muscle known to be supplied by that nerve root is put into antigravity position and tested against external resistance. For example, to test the C5 and C6 spinal motor nerve roots, the examiner would say, "Hold your arms up like this please," and demonstrate the position by abducting his arms laterally to 90 degrees; the patient contracts the deltoids against gravity by abducting both arms laterally to 90 degrees and maintaining that position. The examiner would then say, "Now keep holding them up and don't let me push them down," and apply pressure downward.

Below is a table of muscles I commonly test, with their corresponding peripheral nerves and spinal motor nerve roots:

Table 2.

Action	Muscle	Nerve	Roots
Arm abd. at shoulder	Deltoid	Axillary	C5, C6
Wrist ext. & hand abd.	Ext. carpi radialis	Radial	C5, C6
Wrist flexion & hand abd.	Flexor carpi radialis	Median	C6, C7
Flexion at distal IP joints	Flexor dig. profundus	Median	C7, C8
Finger abduction	Dorsal interossei, ADM	Ulnar	C8, T1
Hip flexion	Iliopsoas	Femoral	L1-L3
Knee extension	Quadriceps	Femoral	L2-L4
Toe dorsiflexion	Ext.hallucis longus	Deep peroneal	L5, S1
Foot dorsiflexion	Tibialis anterior	Deep peroneal	L4, L5
Foot plantar flexion	Gastroc/Soleus	Tibial nerve	S1, S2

Chiropractic Examination

All chiropractors have their own preferred spinal assessment, but all chiropractic examinations would most probably include a postural exam, spinal palpation (which can be incorporated into the palpation portion of the examination), leg length analysis, and any other technique analyses you wish to apply. Record your findings in the chart.

Examination Flow

No-fault clinics can be busy places, with high daily patient volumes. Chiropractors often find that they need to work quickly in order to keep up, and new patient evaluations require more time. Of course, examination quality should never be compromised or sacrificed, but there are ways to structure the examination to make it flow more efficiently. I have found that by organizing the components of the examination to necessitate minimal changes in position by both patient and doctor, the process is streamlined, saving time and patient discomfort.

Here is the typical exam flow I use when examining new patients:

(Greet patient & seat for interview)

Observation and History > Vitals>

(Ask patient to stand before transferring to table)

> Postural exam > Lumbar ROM (all planes) > Patient stands on heels and toes for 3 sec (assesses foot dorsi—and plantar flexion and balance)>

(Ask patient to sit on table. Stand behind patient)

> Cervical ROM (all planes) > Palpation (full spine) > Cervical ortho tests (compression, distraction, shoulder depression, etc.) > Kemp's test>

(Move to stand in front of patient)

> Upper extremity motor (insert shoulder exam if indicated), sensory, and reflex exam > patellar & Achilles reflexes > seated SLR or Bechterew's > Lower extremity motor (resisted knee extension, ankle dorsi/plantar flexion, and hip flexion) > Lower extremity sensory exam >

(Ask patient to lie supine)

> Straight leg raise (and Braggard's) > assess hamstring tightness > FABER

(Ask patient to turn prone)

> Chiropractic exam

Of course, you may fine-tune this grouping to best suit your particular exam style and clinic setup, and there will always be those patients whose examinations will be more complex and require spending more time on a certain component. However, I've found that this general arrangement works most efficiently overall.

Malingering

Recall that earlier, we discussed the nature of the no-fault industry and its symbiosis with personal-injury lawyers and the practice of case "buildup". Attorneys cannot bring an action in court unless there is "serious" injury and costs exceed the benefits provided for under Article 51. Therefore, there is an incentive for claimants to fabricate or exaggerate complaints and injuries to increase the number, type, and costs of treatments in order to reach and exceed that threshold.

It doesn't always happen, but sometimes patients will present for an initial visit with fabricated or exaggerated complaints. You may get a "vibe" from them as they enter the room, or as you take their history and the details of the accident.

Malingering and exaggeration are difficult to "prove" conclusively because pain is subjective. Patients can "game" the exam by giving untruthful responses on the sensory assessment, by giving submaximal effort on motor strength testing and by deliberately limiting their range of motion. Fortunately, you know a little more about anatomy and orthopaedics than they do, and there are assessment procedures you can use that can clarify your "vibes", whenever you get them.

We mentioned Waddell's signs earlier. However, Waddell stated that the signs are only a crude assessment that indicates psychological overlay, are open to misinterpretation, and should not be considered malingering tests.[42] Also, Waddell discourages conveying to patients the impression, in any case, that their symptoms are suspect as this can cause real psychological distress to patients and can aggravate actual symptoms, because individual pain is, in fact, subjective.[43]

There are some so-called malingering tests that I do not recommend using. Mankopf's test calls for aggravating a patient's pain while checking their pulse for an increase over ten beats per minute. This is not really practical in the no-fault setting. Also, Burns' Bench test, which calls for a patient kneeling on a low table to lean over and touch the floor, doesn't seem like something most people without pain can do (try it) and will definitely cause pain in an acute sprain/strain situation where many muscles and soft tissues are inflamed. Some malingering tests out there are specific for radicular pain and may be false positive when soft tissues are inflamed, and everything hurts.

Below are a few malingering tests I like, that you can easily incorporate into your examination procedures.

Hoover's Test: the patient lies supine with the examiner's hands cupped underneath each heel. The patient is asked to raise each leg. If the patient is exerting genuine effort in the presence of pain, the examiner will feel some downward pressure from the leg not being raised. An absence of counter

---

[42] Main CJ, Waddell G (1998) Behavioral Responses to Examination: A Reappraisal of the Interpretation of "Nonorganic Signs". Spine (Phila Pa 1976) 23(21): 2367-2371.

[43] Waddell G. The Back Pain Revolution. 2nd ed. Edinburgh: Churchill Livingstone; 2004. Overreaction should be dropped as it is prone to observer bias and unreliability.

pressure suggests a lack of effort by the patient. This is a good test to use immediately following a straight leg raise.

Distracted Leg Raise: this was discussed earlier. It is the same as the seated leg raise, done while distracting the patient with a patellar reflex or a knee exam.

Heel Tap: the patient sits on the table with hips and knees flexed at 90 degrees. The examiner suggests to the patient that the test may cause pain in the lower back, and then lightly taps the heel with a hand or a reflex hammer. A sudden report of pain in the lower back is a positive test.

O'Donoghue's Test: assess passive vs. active ranges of motion. In patients with pain and true pathology, passive range of motion should be greater than active ROM. The test is considered positive if the patient has less passive than active ROM.

Gordon-Welberry Toe Test: the patient lies supine with the examiner holding the patient's knees and hips flexed to 90 degrees. The examiner flexes the 4th and 5th toes and asks if that does anything to aggravate the patient's back pain. A positive test is a report of back pain. The test can also be done with the ankle.

Pallesthesia: this is loss of vibration sense. Vibration is conducted through the bone to broad areas and should not be confined to a single dermatome. Injury to a single nerve root should not affect vibration perception. A reported loss of vibration sense that is not accompanied by other signs of a general neurological disorder is a positive test.

Bowlus and Currier Test: this is a distraction test to assess the consistency of reported sensory changes in the forearms and hands. Sometime after sensation has been tested once, have the patient invert and cross their arms and test sensation again. If the reported sensory findings are different from the initial results, the test is considered positive.

The Pen Drop Test: this is a distraction test of my own invention. When the patient enters the room, or sometime during the visit, hand the patient a pen on the pretext of some paperwork and "accidentally" drop it at his or her feet. Note if the patient helpfully bends down to get it, and their range of motion. It can also be done with a reflex hammer or any other object. I have actually used this test on occasion, with positive results.

A single positive test should not be considered significant. Also, never confront a patient with positive results to these tests. If you truly suspect that a patient's complaints are fabricated or grossly exaggerated, simply tailor your treatment plan accordingly, or you can always refer the patient to receive physical therapy alone.

11

IMAGING

Just about every patient entering a clinic after an automobile accident will have some form of imaging ordered—usually magnetic resonance imaging (MRI). Patients who are not candidates for MRI (magnetic metal implants or orthopedic hardware, older pacemakers etc.) or those who need bone-specific detail will have computed tomography (CT) exams ordered. Plain film radiography is probably the least utilized imaging modality when it comes to no-fault. Virtually no clinics (or chiropractic practices) that I have seen in the last ten or fifteen years have an in-house x-ray unit. It costs too much to run and maintain, some patients will already have had plain films in the Emergency Department if they went there, and most patients are eventually going to have more advanced imaging anyway. If plain film x-rays are ever deemed necessary, they will be referred out to a radiology facility or sent for a CT instead. So for better or for worse, the likelihood is that you will never shoot or develop a plain film radiograph in no-fault practice. (Personally, I find that unfortunate. The first no-fault clinic I worked in for three years had a unit, and I can remember taking all the different providers' plain films, from skulls to metatarsals and everything in between. With units being too cost-ineffective and too impractical to maintain, roentgenography is sadly becoming a disappearing skill among DCs.) However, there may well be patients in whom there are indications that plain films are indicated, and in these cases, absolutely refer out for them.

Indications and Contraindications for Plain X-Ray

For chiropractors, in the context of a no-fault clinic, there will be certain patients for whom plain x-rays of the cervical spine should definitely be ordered. Those include patients over age 50, those involved car accidents at speeds of over 30 mph, and those who have had transient loss of consciousness.[44]

Contraindications for x-ray are pregnancy, infants, recent high dose radiation exposure, morbid obesity and positioning difficulty (the latter two would reduce image quality and might cause an increased radiation dose to get a better image). Furthermore, for many patients who have had trauma, such as an automobile accident, but are stable and alert without neurological signs or symptoms, cervical plain films may not be necessary and can be deferred.[45]

---

[44] French, SD et al. Risk management for Chiropractors and osteopaths: imaging guidelines for conditions commonly seen in practice. Australasian Chiro & Osteo 2003;11(2)43 .

[45] Hoffman JR, Mower WR, Wolfson AB, Todd KH, Zucker MI. Validity of a set of clinical criteria to rule out injury to the cervical spine in patients with blunt trauma. National Emergency X-Radiography Study Group. N Eng J Med 2000; 343:94-9.

Indications for plain lumbar spine films among patients in a no-fault clinic would be:[46]

- Recent trauma
- Over age 50
- History of malignancy
- History suggesting osteoporosis
- Long term corticosteroid use

There are people who present to no-fault clinics who have had organ transplants (and are on steroids), who have had bouts with cancer, and who are over age 50. Plain films should be strongly considered in this demographic.

MRI

As mentioned, almost every patient in a no-fault clinic will have an MRI ordered of their spinal area of complaint. This, despite the fact that MRIs have not been shown to improve outcome or affect treatment in most cases.[47] Nevertheless, MRIs following automobile accidents have become standard in no-fault clinics, and in addition to providing clinical information, also serve a medicolegal purpose, to document the extent of the injury sustained. Often it will not fall to the DC to order the studies—the MD or PA may do it if they see the patient first—but sometimes it may.

Most MRI facilities will not perform spinal MRIs before 4 weeks have elapsed from the date of the accident, and insurance carriers will usually not reimburse for studies

---

[46] *Supra* 44, at 45

[47] Modic MT, Obuchowski NA, Ross JS, et al. Acute low back pain and radiculopathy: MR imaging findings and their prognostic role and effect on outcome. Radiology. 2005;237(2):597—604.

performed earlier than that. This is because various guidelines suggest that MRI before 4-6 weeks is unlikely to alter treatment decisions or outcomes.[48] In many clinics, providers will order the MRIs at the initial visit anyway. However, in my opinion, if you as the chiropractor are expected to order the MRIs, it is preferable to wait until the patient has had 2-3 weeks of treatment and therapy before ordering MRIs.

Also, because most patients see the chiropractor several times per week, as opposed to the 1-2 times per month they see the MD or PA who may have ordered the study, they often ask the DC what the results of the MRIs are, and to explain the findings to them. Spinal MRIs are usually concerned with disc findings, so a review of the nomenclature[49] concerning disc findings is worthwhile.

Normal Disc—a normal disc consists of an outer annulus and inner nucleus. The disc is within the disc space boundaries, which are the endplates and the outer apophyseal edges of the vertebrae above and below.

Bulge—a disc is considered "bulging" when it extends beyond the edges of the vertebral ring apophyses, around the entire circumference of the disc. It occurs when there are tears in the annulus, but it is not considered a herniation. Bulges can be asymmetric when they extend more than 25% beyond the apophysis on one side. Bulges are often asymptomatic and therefore probably not clinically significant. In one study,

---

[48] Gilbert F, Grant A, Gillan M, et al. Scottish Back Trial Group. Low back pain: influence of early MR imaging or CT on treatment and outcome—multicenter randomized trial. Radiology. 2004;231:343-51

[49] Fardon DF, Williams AL, Dohring EJ, Murtagh FR, Rothman SLG & Sze GK. Lumbar disc nomenclature: version 2.0: recommendations of the combined task forces of the North American Spine Society, the American Society of Spine Radiology and the American Society of Neuroradiology. The Spine Journal, 2014:14(11), 2525-2545.

slightly more than half of asymptomatic subjects had one or two disc bulges.[50]

Annular Fissure—this is a separation between annular fibers that does not extend beyond the exterior of the annulus. Think of it as an interior "crack."

Herniation—a focal displacement of nuclear material that extends beyond the limits of the disc space boundary and is less than 25% of disc circumference. It can be contained (covered) by the outer annulus, or uncontained.

Protrusion—in a protrusion, the distance between the edges of the herniated material is greater at the base of the herniation (closer to the disc) that at the apex (furthest from the disc).

Extrusion—a disc is extruded when the edges of the herniated material are narrower at the portion closer to the disc than at the portion furthest from it.

Migration—indicates displacement of the herniated material extending away from the disc it herniated from.

Sequestration—the herniated material has separated from the disc it has herniated from.

Intravertebral Herniation—a herniation in the Y axis; also known as a Schmorl's node.

---

[50] Jensen MC, Brant-Zawadzki MN, Obuchowski N, Modic MT, Malkasian D, Ross JS. Magnetic resonance imaging of the lumbar spine in people without back pain. New England Journal of Medicine. 1994 Jul 14;331(2):69-73.

Disc findings are also described by their localization:

Central—herniations usually occur slightly right or left of center, since the posterior longitudinal ligament (PLL) is thickest in this area.

Sub-articular—this is the area below the facet joints, and is the most common area of disc herniation, since the PLL is thinner here.

Foraminal—the herniation occurs directly into the intervertebral foramen (IVF). These are not as common as many believe—only 5-10% of herniations occur in this location, which is probably why most patients with disc herniation do not have classic radicular symptoms and findings.

Patients are often anxious to know what their MRI study shows. It's important to put the findings in perspective for the patient and explain that an MRI is only a picture—a "snapshot" of anatomy; it cannot give any information about function, and MRI findings do not always correlate with clinical findings[51] or predict outcomes.[52] It is helpful to explain that MRI is only part of the diagnostic "picture." I always explain that we treat the patient, not the MRI report.

---

[51] Boden SD, Davis DO, Dina TS, Patronas NJ, Wiesel SW. Abnormal magnetic-resonance scans of the lumbar spine in asymptomatic subjects. A prospective investigation.J. Bone Joint Surg. Am. 72:403-408, 1990.

[52] McNee P, Shambrook J, Harris EC, Kim M, Sampson M, Palmer KT, Coggon D. Predictors of long-term pain and disability in patients with low back pain investigated by magnetic resonance imaging: a longitudinal study. BMC musculoskeletal disorders. 2011 Oct 14;12(1):234.

As a chiropractor, it's important to understand this as well; *MRI findings are not destiny.* Patients can and do recover—it just takes time. It's important to convey this to patients so that they do not lapse into self-reinforcing pain behaviors.[53]

---

[53] Hadjistavropoulos, Thomas, et al. "Biopsychosocial Approaches to Pain." *Pain: Psychological Perspectives*, Psychology Press, 2013, pp. 49–53.

12

OTHER TESTING

EMG

Aside from imaging, no-fault clinics also provide other testing of relevance to chiropractors. One of the most commonly utilized tests is the electrodiagnostic study, or electromyography (EMG).

The EMG, which also includes a nerve conduction velocity (NCV) study, is used to assess the integrity of the peripheral nerves and the spinal nerve roots by recording the conduction velocity of an impulse sent along the nerve, and by recording electrical signals in muscles known to be supplied by a specific nerve root.

The NCV portion is split into upper and lower extremity regions, testing sensory and motor nerves in both. In the upper extremity portion, sensory and motor divisions of the median, ulnar, and radial nerves are tested (some omit radial motor), and in the lower extremity, the peroneal (motor), superficial peroneal (sensory), tibial (motor), and sural (sensory) nerves are tested. The examiner affixes surface electrodes at specified points on the tested limb, and with an electrical stimulator connected to the testing machine, fires a small electrical impulse along the nerve (millivolts for motor, microvolts for sensory) to reference and recording electrodes from specific locations. The computer calculates the average velocity of that impulse using the time taken for the impulse to travel and the known distances between the stimulation points and the reference electrode. The recorded velocities and other parameters are compared to normal values.

The NCV component is often used in the diagnosis of carpal tunnel syndrome, where it is both highly sensitive and specific, taking nerve conduction velocity measurements across the wrist. In other diagnostic uses, it is sensitive but not as specific.[54]

The electromyographic portion is performed by inserting needle electrodes into specific muscles known to be supplied by specific spinal nerve roots, and observing for and/or recording any abnormal pathological electrical activity that would indicate denervation of the muscle related to injury at the nerve root. It can also be used to assess severity, localization, and prognosis of a nerve injury. It is mainly used in the no-fault setting to assess for the presence of radiculopathy. Electromyography is highly operator-dependent—meaning the skill of the electromyographer is important—and the EMG findings must be observed and interpreted in real time.

EMG and NCV testing is usually not performed until several weeks following an injury. This is because it usually

---

[54] LaJoie AS, McCabe SJ, Thomas B, Edgell SE. Determining the sensitivity and specificity of common diagnostic tests for carpal tunnel syndrome using latent class analysis. Plastic and reconstructive surgery. 2005 Aug 1;116(2):502-7.

takes this long for Wallerian degeneration in injured nerve axons (depending on the length of the axon) to manifest as decreased motor unit recruitment in supplied muscle, although a skilled electromyographer can detect changes as early as one week.[55]

Both the EMG and NCV tests are somewhat unpleasant. The multiple electrical stimulations feel like a strong "static shock" one might feel after walking barefoot on carpet, and the needle electrodes can be painful as well.

In the no-fault setting it is usually the medical physician who performs the needle EMG, but in New York State chiropractors with proper certification may perform these as well, and recently many chiropractors have been doing so. I received EMG certification after training daily with a neurologist for a year and spent another two years performing NCV and EMG testing in various offices, including no-fault. In my experience (and corroborated with other EMG physician colleagues), while abnormalities on NCV are not that unusual, true radicular EMG findings are relatively less common.

As with imaging studies, patients will sometimes ask the chiropractor to explain the results to them. Fortunately, the results are usually tabulated on a printed report. As with imaging studies, the results should always be taken in clinical context, and treatment is geared toward the patient, not the test result.

Computerized ROM

Many no-fault clinics bring in technicians to perform computerized range-of-motion analyses. This test involves placement of a dual computerized inclinometer on different

---

[55] Feinberg J. EMG: myths and facts. HSS Journal. 2006 Feb 1;2(1):19-21.

points on the patient's spine and having them perform various movements throughout a range of motion.

Computerized ROM testing provides objective data that can be very useful in monitoring clinical progress from baseline; the patient is tested at the beginning of treatment and subsequently every 10 days or so, in some clinics. It is useful from a medicolegal standpoint to quantify progression, or lack thereof (keeping in mind, of course, that any ROM evaluation can be "gamed" if the patient is intent on doing so). Also, ROM assessments are most reliable when the patient is tested with the same examiner and device.[56]

As with EMG, chiropractors are not usually the ones performing these tests, although they theoretically may, and the results are usually available to review in the patient's chart should the interest arise.

---

[56] Mannion AF, Klein GN, Dvorak J, Lanz C. Range of global motion of the cervical spine: intraindividual reliability and the influence of measurement device. European Spine Journal. 2000 Oct 1;9(5):379-85.

13

DIAGNOSIS & TREATMENT

Diagnosis

Once you have examined the patient and reviewed any imaging (or while awaiting results), you must establish a diagnosis for the patient, and record it in the chart using the ICD-10 system. (Appendix D of this book includes a list of the most commonly used ICD-10 codes by chiropractors in no-fault practice.) The most common and most frequently recorded diagnoses in no-fault clinics, unsurprisingly, include cervical, thoracic, and lumbar sprains and strains, ligamentous injury, cervical and lumbosacral pain, disc displacement and herniation, and headaches.

Proper and accurate diagnosis and coding are important; not just for the obvious, clinical reasons, but also because the diagnosis is submitted to a third-party payor and is the basis for reimbursement. A pattern of intentional inaccuracies in coding could conceivably attract the kind of authoritative attention, and consequences, that we talked about in Chapters 5 & 6. Nobody wants that.

Probably the most common inaccuracy in diagnosis I have seen in no-fault clinics involves the misapplied code for radiculopathy. Radiculopathy is a clinical phenomenon; the Medline dictionary defines radiculopathy as "irritation of or injury to a nerve root (as from being compressed) that typically causes pain, numbness, or weakness in the part of the body which is supplied with nerves from that root."[57] In order for a diagnosis of radiculopathy to apply, a patient must complain of radiating *pain, numbness* (or paresthesia), or exhibit *weakness* in a limb or body part supplied by that nerve root. However, I have frequently seen this code utilized for patients who complained only of local back and/or neck pain, without any extremity radiation, numbness, or weakness.

This is, of course, inaccurate. Only patients who complain of *radicular* symptoms, or have *radicular* signs or evidence should be given a diagnosis of *radiculopathy*. If they only have local spinal pain and findings (as a great many patients do), there are plenty of other codes that can cover that.

Diagnoses can be updated (and should be) when new diagnostic evidence becomes available. If the patient complains only of local neck pain at their initial visit and has no positive radicular orthopedic tests, no code for radiculopathy should be applied. If two weeks later, the patient begins to complain of numbness and tingling in their thumb and index finger, you would re-examine the patient. If a shoulder depression test reproduces the symptoms, you could then update their diagnosis. If an EMG test finds evidence of a radiculopathy, it would also be appropriate to update the diagnosis as such. A disc herniation, however, in

---

[57] "Radiculopathy": http://c.merriam-webster.com/medlineplus/radiculopathy. Accessed September 2017.

the absence of any related clinical findings, is not sufficient to support a diagnosis of radiculopathy; we have already established that disc findings and symptoms are poorly correlated.

I'm not sure why this miscoding is so prevalent; is it simple misunderstanding, or is it done with the belief that certain diagnoses are associated with longer periods of treatment reimbursement by the insurance carrier? Either way, routine misapplication of diagnosis codes can invite increased scrutiny, such as records audits and EUOs. If you or a patient for whom you submitted a diagnosis of radiculopathy are called to an EUO, and a savvy examiner asks if they had any radicular symptoms and the answer is no, and there is no evidence in the chart to support the diagnosis (or the diagnosis was submitted prior to the date of the evidence), that's materially false information— the carrier can deny the entire claim retroactively. Can it then also begin a lookback at all your other claims for similar "inaccuracies" and misapplied diagnoses and request repayment of their reimbursements? Don't think it's impossible; in an environment that is saturated with fraud, where insurance companies are looking to conserve every dollar, such tactics are certainly not beyond the realm of possibility.

A full treatment of diagnosis coding for billing purposes is beyond the scope of this book, but there are many fine publications available for that purpose.

Treatment Plan

Once the diagnosis has been established and it is deemed safe to do so, treatment can begin. But first, you need a plan of care, which should include visit frequency, technique, prognosis, goals, and a re-evaluation point, all specifically tailored for the patient.

Typically, a patient coming in for a routine visit will go to the therapy area where they will be shown to a curtained "bay," and lie on a table while the therapist applies electrical stimulation, heat or ice, massage and other therapies. This is usually directly followed by the acupuncturist's treatment, which includes needling and sometimes moxibustion or "cupping." Finally, if the patient has not already done so beforehand, they will now go see the chiropractor.

As was discussed in earlier chapters, no-fault clinics are designed so that chiropractors generally do one thing: adjust the spine. (Some would argue that that's all that chiropractors do anywhere—but that's a discussion for a different book.) Any modalities (electrical muscle stimulation, etc.), or therapeutic exercises are supposed to be done with the patient by the physical therapist. In many clinics, however, I have found that at least when it comes to the spine, PTs are not addressing active rehab with patients. In most clinics, spinal rehab consists of basically having the patient lie prone with stim, heat, and acupuncture needles in their back for 45 minutes. So chiropractors should pay some attention to not only adjusting, but also active rehabilitation.

As all chiropractors know, there are many adjustment techniques to choose from when adjusting the spine, and many chiropractors have certain techniques or styles that they prefer. I'm not a technique "expert," and will not presume to tell anyone that any particular technique is "better" than any other, but I would maintain that some techniques are going to be better for certain patients and/or situations than others. Not every technique is going to be the best approach for every patient, or at every point in the course of treatment. For example, when it comes to Diversified adjusting, patients are often in acute pain and spasm close to their accident dates, and may not be able to tolerate a Diversified-type adjustment with an audible release. Some patients may be apprehensive. Some may be too large to comfortably and effectively adjust. Some may have other injuries or comorbidities that preclude

Diversified adjusting—like rib, clavicle, and other fractures, or patients on anticoagulants with stroke history, to name a few.

Having several techniques to choose from gives you the tools to be able to see patients with a wider variety of conditions more effectively. It's always good to have as many tools in your "bag of tricks" as you can. Let's examine a few technique approaches and their application in the no-fault setting.

Diversified

This is most chiropractors' "bread and butter" technique, but I have found that in more than a few no-fault clinics, chiropractors are not using it to adjust patients; I often used Diversified in many offices where I did coverage, and patients there would tell me that their regular chiropractor had never adjusted them that way before. Perhaps some chiropractors are concerned with liability, and would rather use low or non-force techniques to keep the chance of any adverse reaction low. Maybe some chiropractors feel that patients wouldn't like Diversified adjusting, and would rather use a lower or non-force technique to avoid "scaring" patients away and losing their revenue. Or, maybe it's just easier to see 40-plus patients a day when you're using an instrument. I'm not saying that Diversified should be used exclusively, of course. But I recall covering one doctor in a no fault clinic who used only an Arthrostim instrument (an automatic impulse adjusting tool) and specifically told me *not* to do anything else.

It's okay to use Diversified. Obviously, like with any other technique, patients need to be selected appropriately; it's not necessarily for everybody, or for every visit. But for thepatients with whom it can be safely and comfortably used, the effects are wonderful, and patients are highly appreciative.

It's okay not to use Diversified. There will be patients who are not candidates for Diversified. Patients who have a history of stroke, who are taking anticoagulant medications, who have severe degenerative changes with sharp osteophytes, rib or other spinal fractures, and who have had one or more spinal levels fused or fixated with hardware are among those who should not receive high velocity, low amplitude (HVLA) manipulation adjusting to relevant regions.

There are also patients who are not ready for Diversified adjusting *yet*, or who would be as well or better served by using a different technique; other techniques also get effective results. Patients in acute pain, with severely restricted ROM and muscle spasm, will often not tolerate manipulative adjustment techniques and may get scared off any further chiropractic treatment if they experience pain during treatment. I have found it is better to use gentle manual mobilization techniques in the early phase of care with patients in severe pain and spasm and incorporate manipulation once the patient is better able to tolerate it.

Instrument Adjusting

Manual manipulation is not always an option. Some older patients have osteoporosis,[58] or are fearful of manipulation that produces audible cavitation ("cracking"). A patient may be unable to lie in position to be adjusted manually or may have personal issues regarding touch.[59] For these patients, instrument adjustment can be a good alternative. There are

---

[58] Cooperstein R, Killinger LZ. Chiropractic techniques in the care of the geriatric patient. In: Gleberzon BJ, editor. Chiropractic care of the older patient. First Ed. Oxford, UK: Butterworth-Heinemann; 2001. pp. 359–383.

[59] Gleberzon BJ. Chiropractic Name Techniques in Canada: A continued look at demographic trends and their impact on issues of jurisprudence. J Can Chiro Assoc. 2002;46(4):241–256

many types and brands of chiropractic adjustment instruments available, including the Activator ™ series of instruments, the Impulse,™ the ArthroStim,™ and generic instruments. Personally, I have always found using a generic instrument to be adequate; one need not subscribe to a particular "branded" technique system to achieve good results. If you're a doctor who usually adjusts with manual Diversified technique, it may seem unlikely that simply using an instrument on the spine could be effective. However, many studies have shown that instrument adjusting modulates and reduces pain[60] and improves segmental motion in the spine by affecting muscle spindle response to mechanoreceptors.[61] Plus, a lot of patients actually seem to like it.

Flexion Table

Flexion is an effective low-velocity and low-force technique approach, particularly for patients with lower back pain from disc symptoms, and has been shown to have better outcomes than active trunk exercises in chronic low back pain.[62] Personally, having practiced with and without one, I have found that a flexion table is invaluable in a no-fault office. Many patients have moderate to severe lower back pain, and many patients are also morbidly overweight, making side-posture adjusting less practical. Flexion (manual

---

[60] Song XJ, Gan Q, Cao JL, Wang ZB, Rupert RL. Spinal manipulation reduces pain and hyperalgesia after lumbar intervertebral foramen inflammation in the rat. Journal of manipulative and physiological therapeutics. 2006 Jan 31;29(1):5-13.

[61] Reed WR, Pickar JG, Sozio RS, Liebschner MA, Little JW, Gudavalli MR. Characteristics of Paraspinal Muscle Spindle Response to Mechanically Assisted Spinal Manipulation: A Preliminary Report. Journal of Manipulative and Physiological Therapeutics. 2017 Jul 1;40(6):371-80.

[62] Gudavalli MR, Cambron JA, McGregor M, et al. A randomized clinical trial and subgroup analysis to compare flexion–distraction with active exercise for chronic low back pain. European Spine Journal. 2006;15(7):1070-1082. doi:10.1007/s00586-005-0021-8.

or mechanical) can be employed in treating these patients to great benefit. It can be used while the doctor applies a Cox-type technique—securing the patient's legs with a strap and stabilizing supra-adjacent vertebrae with one hand to isolate traction at a particular disc level. Or, the table can simply move automatically, which effects a gentle oscillating mobilization that many patients find soothing.

Pelvic Blocking

Especially if you don't have a flexion table, pelvic blocking techniques can be very useful when treating patients with lower back and sciatic symptoms who are not candidates for manual manipulation. A manual modified Cox-type distraction and mobilization technique can also be used while the patient is on the blocks, and I have found this very useful in some cases of lower back pain where manipulation was not an option and no flexion table was available.

Complicated Cases

Many chiropractors are familiar with what is known in the profession as the "80-10-10 rule"; this bit of professional folk wisdom states that of a given set of patients in a chiropractic practice, 80% will improve completely, 10% will improve only partially, and 10% will not improve at all, or get worse and require referral.

While those exact percentages may not be accurate, the general proportions of this rule seem to hold out in practice. No-fault clinics are not very different in this respect. Most patients do improve, although it can be slow, often many months. Some patients, unfortunately, develop chronic pain patterns that do not vary much, even after 6 months of multiple medical and chiropractic treatment approaches. And then there are the patients who not only aren't getting better but need drastic intervention. It can be easy to become inured to patients' complaints in a no-fault clinic—after all, everyone there is complaining of pain, every visit. But if we're not vigilant, seemingly routine cases of non-improvement can devolve into serious problems that can have lasting consequences. The following case study illustrates how being clinically "on your toes" (no pun intended) can mean the difference between a better outcome and an adverse one.

Case Study

The following case is real; the name and other identifying data have been changed to protect privacy, although the patient gave permission to relate her case. It's an example of a case where careful, regular observation and re-evaluation, and not just treating on autopilot, made the difference in outcome. The case notes are recreated below; the initial exam is expanded, with much of it as originally written, and the daily SOAP notes are recreated verbatim.

Patient name: _____Jessica R._____ Age: __41__

Date of accident: __March 14__ Date of exam: __March 20__

History:

The patient is a 41 yo female restrained driver struck on the driver's side. No head trauma or LOC reported. Transported by ambulance to East Brooklyn Hospital where MRI scans of the cervical and lumbar spine were taken (attached).

Past History:

None

Current Complaints:

Pt c/o diffuse H/A 5/10, local dull neck pain bilaterally 6/10, & 10/10 intense LBP rad to Lt. leg. C/O difficulty walking, difficulty sitting (L antalgic lean). Weakness esp L leg

Gait:

Guarded—L antalgic lean—marked

ROM (Observed)

Cervical Spine

Flexion 20   L Rotation 40   L Lateral Flexion 10

Extension 0   R Rotation 40   R Lateral Flexion 10

Lumbar Spine

Flexion 0   L Rotation 0   L Lateral Flexion 0

Extension 0   R Rotation 0   R Lateral Flexion 0

–All ROM with pain

Tenderness & spasm palp at bilat upper trap, C/S & L/S paraspinals, L/S jct and QL. Marked spasm L/S.

Cervical Distraction +   Cervical Distraction +

Shoulder Depression +   Valsalva Maneuver +

Kemp's Test +   Straight Leg Raise + *

*seated—exam limited due to severe patient discomfort.

Motor Exam:

U/E motor 5/5 bilat deltoid, wrist & finger flex/ext

L/E motor—Pt able to walk Heel & toe, w/ pain in L foot on L ankle dorsiflexion

Sensory Exam:

No hyper/hypo sensation U/E or L/E

Reflexes:

DTRs +2/+2 bilat at knee, ankle, wrist, elbow

CN II-XII grossly normal

Impression:

C/S sprain/strain and derangement, L/S radiculitis

Plan:

Tx to C/S only to include light C/S mobiliz, progressing to C/S CMT as tolerated—re-eval in 2 wks. Pt adv to continue PT & use ice @ home on L/S 10 min qh.

As you can see, this patient was in severe lower back pain with radiating left leg pain. This was a true radiculitis; she had zero range of motion in any plane in her lumbar spine. She couldn't even bend her trunk enough to sit on the table. To test her knee and ankle reflexes, I had to take her to another exam room that had a medical exam table, which was higher, and which I thought would be easier for her to get onto. (It wasn't. She was literally in tears.)

This was six days following her accident. My plan, since she also had neck pain and stiffness that was not radicular, was to treat her neck while letting her receive passive modalities (ice, electrical stimulation) in physical therapy, and then revisit her lumbar spine in two weeks.

Several days later her hospital MRI reports were sent over:

MRI LUMBAR SPINE WO CONTRAST- Details

Narrative
Diagnosis: Disc herniation, low back pain, weakness of the lower extremity

Sagittal T1, proton-density, T2-weighted and fat-suppressed T2-weighted images as well as axial proton density and T2-weighed images were obtained.

At L5-S1, there is a disc herniation with a superiorly extruded fragment that measures approximately 11mm from superior to inferior, 8mm from left to right and 7mm from anterior to posterior. This is best demonstrated on the sagittal images and axial images 18 through 20.

There are mild degenerative changes of the intervertebral disc at L4-L5 with a tiny focal central disc herniation is best demonstrated on the midline sagittal images and axial image 16. The remaining intervertebral discs appear normal. The vertebrae maintain normal signal, configuration, and alignment. There is no evidence of fracture, subluxation or focal bone lesion. There is no epidural disease. The conus demonstrates normal morphology and signal and is not compressed.

Impression

---

1. Left paracentral herniation with a superiorly extruded disc fragment at L5-S1.
2. Degenerative changes with a tiny central disc herniation at L4-L5.
3. No compression of the distal spinal cord or conus.

Well, that certainly explains why she was having radicular pain, doesn't it? But her initial neuro exam was basically normal; she had lower extremity reflexes, and she could walk on her heels and toes. She would get PT and pain meds from the MD, and hopefully the inflammation and pain would subside. As a chiropractor, sometimes the only thing you can do for a patient is . . . nothing. This patient couldn't even get onto the table, let alone tolerate an adjustment.

Below are the handwritten portions of my notes (they were combination check-off notes, so that data is not shown here) as treatment progressed, recreated exactly as written.

March 22 (second visit, 3 days post-injury)

Pt still c/o severe L/S pain—amb w/ a L antalgic lean. Flexion w/ L lat flexion attempted, but d/c d/t pt discomfort. Recommend PT L/S only for next 1-2 wks to allow for pain level to subside.

The patient was in a lot of pain and desperately wanted to try something; we agreed I would try using flexion technique, with lateral flexion to relieve pressure from the disc. However, she could not tolerate that either and it was stopped.

March 28 (third visit, 8 days post-injury)

Cont to c/o LBP—walks w/ guarded gait & R antalgia. States she has an LSO & it is helpful. C/O sore neck 'kink' & stiffness. CMT c/s only supine. Well tolerated.

I had advised her to get herself a lumbar support belt, which she was wearing and said that it helped. We continued working with her neck only.

March 29 (fourth visit, 9 days post-injury)

Pt states pain slightly improving, wearing an LSO @ home. Assmt of bilat EHLs reveals no weakness. CMT c/s only.

At this point, the patient appears to be feeling "slightly" better. I was concerned and watchful enough to have checked her distal motor function again and found no abnormality. Treatment continued this way with chiropractic treatment of the cervical spine only for seven more visits, through the end of April.

On the morning of May 2, her twelfth visit and 42 days post-injury, Jessica limped into my treatment room with a straight cane she had been using for a while. She complained she was still in terrible pain and still having weakness in her left leg, and things didn't seem like they had been getting any better with the physical therapy and medication. In fact, she said, they were getting worse. So I re-examined her.

May 2 (Twelfth visit, 42 days post-injury)

Pt unable to plantar flex L foot or dorsiflex L EHL (1+/5) & there is sensory deficit entire L foot. Pt unsure if surgery has been discussed. Discussed case w/ JM (PA) for poss surgical referral.

I found that she was unable to plantar flex her left foot and only weakly able to extend her left big toe—actions she had no trouble doing 6 weeks earlier. Remember that during the time leading up to this visit, she was under PT care, as well as following up with the physician's assistant. Apparently, no one else had re-examined her, or if they had, they missed this.

I asked the patient if anyone had discussed the possibility of surgery with her. She told me that she had seen an orthopedist, and that he had recommended continuing with therapy, and that he wasn't recommending surgery.

I took the file into the next room to discuss it with the physician's assistant, and she said she would bring it up next time she saw Jessica for a follow-up.

May 10 (Thirteenth visit, 50 days post-injury)

Pt states she saw IME orthopedic surgeon. Spoke w/ Dr. M and he concurred that pt needs to see spinal surgeon, and that a referral will be arranged.

At her next visit over a week later, I joined her follow up visit with the physician assistant. There seemed to be some confusion; the PA was hearing that Jessica had recently seen an orthopedic surgeon, who had advised against surgery. In light of her severe pain and distal motor weakness, though, that didn't make any sense. I questioned Jessica a bit more deeply, and came to realize that what had actually happened was that she had gone to an IME—an Independent Medical Examination—and the orthopedic surgeon there had just told her to continue therapy.

An IME is an examination that the insurance company orders to determine if the patient needs continuing treatment.

The patient will need to see doctors and providers contracted by the insurer, of each type that is treating the patient, who will examine them and determine if they need to continue that particular treatment. The IME doctors are not there to decide *how* the patient should be treated—they do not advocate for the patient and there is no doctor-patient relationship.

If the examiner determines that the patient is not making any more progress, they usually determine that no further treatment is necessary and therefore will not be reimbursed. The examining provider will not tell the patient this at the examination—they will be mailed a written determination within a week—*they will just tell the patient to go back and continue with their therapy.* This is apparently what happened with Jessica . . . and she construed it to mean that she had been examined and told she did not need surgery.

I then spoke with the office's medical director, who agreed with me that based on Jessica's signs and declining motor function, she definitely needed to see a spinal surgeon. Now, we just had to find her one. Usually, even with so many patients in no-fault offices with back pain, disc findings, and other abnormal test results, surgery is rarely needed, and so there usually isn't one "in-house." The staff was not able to make a referral right away, so first I gave her the names of a neurologist and neurosurgeon I had dealt with in the past.

May 11 (Fourteenth visit, 51 days post-injury)

Patient given referral to neurologist / neurosurgeon (WB)

When I checked with the patient over the next several visits, she had still not contacted the neurologist or neurosurgeon I had referred her to, and I urged her to do so.

Finally, she did—and told me that they did not accept no-fault cases. Back to square one.

I contacted a neurologist I used to work with, and he gave me the name of a spine surgeon. When I called his office, his appointment manager said yes, they do accept no-fault cases. However, before they accepted Jessica's case, they needed to review her MRI to see if she was a good surgical candidate. They needed the actual images, not the report—which is all I had.

I spoke to Jessica, who said she would arrange to get the images on disk from the hospital. But over the next several visits, she was frustrated with the hospital bureaucracy and her apparent inability to get through to the right department. She said they wouldn't give it to her without a release, and she said she was getting the runaround. This seemed strange to me, and I wasn't sure if she was subconsciously avoiding the prospect of surgery or if she was caught up in confusing red tape, but regardless I told her I would get the images myself.

I had Jessica sign a records release form and called the hospital's records department, who told me that they would be happy to send a disk to both me and the surgeon's office. Shortly the disk arrived. I had never seen the actual images before—only the report, so I pulled up her lumbar MRI study.

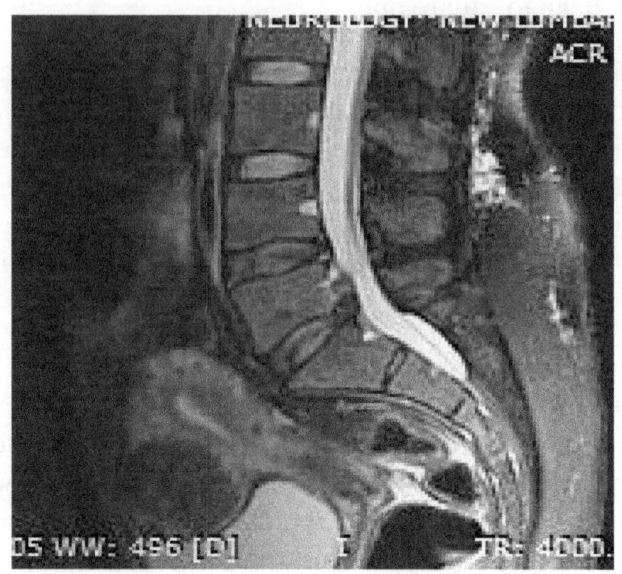
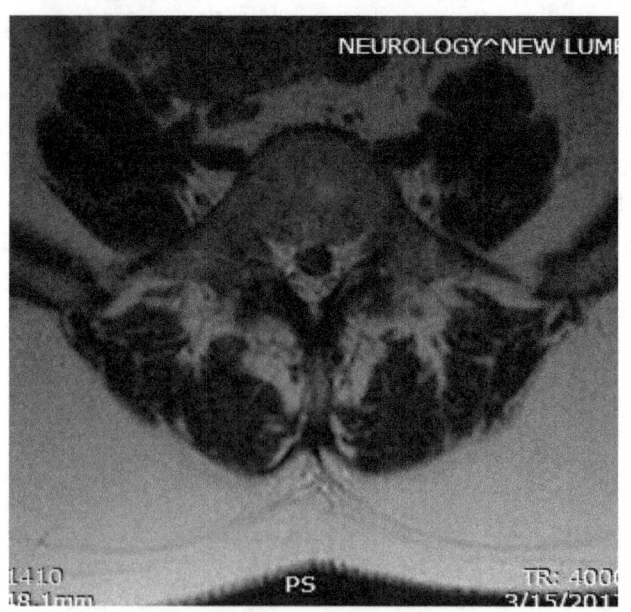

If the MRI report didn't explain why Jessica was having such severe pain and sensory-motor deficit, the images sure did. The superiorly extruded fragment mentioned in the report is clearly visible on the sagittal image. There it was—the cause of all her pain and disability.

May 31 (Eighteenth visit, 73 days post-injury)

** Patient scheduled for spine surgery 6/2 **

Finally, Jessica was scheduled for spine surgery. I called the patient several days later and she said that everything had gone well.

June 15 (Nineteenth visit, two weeks post-surgery, 87 days post-injury)

Pt is s/p 2 wks L/S diskectomy—3" scar midline L4-S1 healing well. Pt has ↑ ROM L/S & is no longer using cane. Pt has dorsiflexion & plantar flexion of L foot & can Heel / toe walk. CMT c/s only.

Two weeks after spine surgery, Jessica was doing well. She was still having some lower back pain, but significantly less than previously. Also, her range of motion had improved, and she was able to walk without limping and had restored distal motor function to her left foot. I continued treating her cervical spine.

This case study underscores the importance of closely monitoring concerning clinical situations, performing regular re-exams, and effective doctor-patient communication. In a clinic with an MD, a PA, and a PT, this patient's deteriorating neurological condition was not picked up by any of them. And I don't necessarily believe it's because they're sloppy—they would have probably noticed it eventually, and I just caught it first. But timing can often mean the difference between a positive outcome and one that's not so good. Also, there was a communication breakdown between Jessica and the clinic providers—she misunderstood the IME process and the nature of the IME doctor's role, and thought the IME doctor was telling her she didn't need surgery. She relayed that to the other providers in our office (neither of us having been aware that she was even going to an IME), who in turn misunderstood Jessica, which also might have delayed the surgery that she needed. It was only further, more probing questioning of Jessica that revealed that the doctor was "from the insurance" and the realization that it was, in fact, an IME. (Why the IME doctor didn't find sensory-motor deficit on his supposedly thorough exam is a whole other question, but knowing what the IME process is like, it isn't that surprising.)

Thankfully, this case has a happy ending; Jessica regained sensory and motor function, her pain level improved tremendously, and she achieved a full recovery.

14

RECORDKEEPING

All practices and practitioners must maintain patient records and chart every patient's clinical progress, and no-fault clinics are no exception. What does seem to be different is that while most medical and chiropractic practices have embraced the digital age and moved to electronic medical records (EMR) and charting systems, no-fault clinics have largely resisted this trend, and still use paper charting systems.

This is most likely for several reasons. First, patients in no-fault clinics generate enormous amounts of paper—intake forms for each practitioner, various no-fault forms, multiple test results for MRIs, EMGs, and ROM tests, outcome questionnaires, other notes, and the list goes on. It's more practical to keep them on paper than spend hours scanning them into electronic format. Also, each practitioner (chiropractor, acupuncturist, other specialists) keeps their own chart system, with separate examination forms, daily progress notes, and test results—especially since they are separate professional business entities under separate P.C.s. Again, it's simpler to maintain records in paper format. Finally, billing for no-fault also somehow still exists in the electronic Stone Age; to my knowledge, billing to no-fault insurance is still done the old-fashioned way—on paper. Since daily progress notes must accompany bills anyway, it is again simpler to just keep everything on paper.

Of course, this makes recordkeeping in no-fault offices all the more cumbersome. Some offices deal with the paper burden well. Other chiropractic no-fault practices that I have seen are sloppy and cut corners with recordkeeping, in both content and format.

Record Format

There was a time, mostly in the mid-70s to mid-90s, when a "travel card" was the charting system that was in vogue in chiropractic offices. (The card was so named because it would "travel" with the patient from the front desk receptionist, who would hand it to the patient to bring it with them back to the doctor, and vice versa on the way out after the visit.) The 8.5 x 11" card was folded in half and was jam-packed full of little boxes and check spaces to record initial palpatory findings, spinal subluxation levels, and other findings on the inside of the card, and had a small column of lines on the outside back for daily notes. On the front was demographic information and three columns to record visit dates and charges. Usually, all that was recorded was the date of the visit. Occasionally a note might be written in the column of lines on the back if an unusual visit occurred. The front had space to record ninety visit dates; often, the travel card was the patient's entire clinical record. Any outside test results like MRIs (not as commonly done 20 and 30 years ago as they are today) were folded in half and slid into the card fold. The only documents kept in an actual file folder in a cabinet were billing statements and correspondence. Obviously, times have changed, and a travel card system is not really adequate for clinical recordkeeping, either in a general practice or a no-fault clinic (although I have seen them in use in at least one, where daily SOAP sheets were folded into the card.)

There are two kinds of chiropractic recordkeeping systems that seem to predominate in no-fault clinics: the file folder and the ring binder. We're all familiar with the file folder—it's been pretty standard for decades in medical and some chiropractic offices. The file folder system varies somewhat from clinic to clinic and by individual practitioner, but basically, within the folder is the patient's completed intake forms and signed consents and releases, an exam report, daily progress notes, and any diagnostic test results. Basically, all the clinical information any practitioner needs to be familiar with the patient's condition and the arc of their care, from the beginning, is there at their fingertips. Any chiropractor seeing the patient can look back and see what the situation was a week or a month in the past.

The ring binder, on the other hand, seems to be something that is unique to no-fault clinics, and something that I've seen mainly in the past 5-10 years. Here's how it works: clinical SOAP notes for each visit (complaint, objective findings, areas adjusted, etc.) are arranged in separate blocks, with 5 blocks on a page. The patient's name is written at the top and that page is placed in the binder alphabetically by last name. When a patient comes in for a visit, the chiropractor opens the binder to that patient's sheet, which they will sign in a designated spot. The doctor will check off the SOAP information for that visit, sign the block, and repeat the procedure with the next patient.

This system is used in some no-fault clinics for a couple of reasons. First, as I mentioned earlier, in many no-fault clinics the chiropractor room is very small—often an 8 by 10 foot (or smaller) room with a small desk, a chair or two, and an adjusting table. There's hardly any room for a file cabinet, and a binder system makes it unnecessary to keep entire patient files in the room to see the patients. Second, when it comes time for billing, it's easy for the billing people to keep up to date—every two weeks the binder is emptied, the sheets copied and sent along with the bills for each date, and the originals (hopefully) placed in the main file folder.

The problem with this system is it leaves the treating chiropractor very much in the dark, records wise. There's no clinical context to the record because there's nothing but the visits on the sheet that is currently in the binder to be a guide—all the previous visits' notes were removed for billing and put in a different folder. The initial examination report is not in there, nor are any imaging or other clinical test results. If a patient comes in who hasn't been in since before the last billing cycle, how are you going to remember anything about what you did last time? I worked covering absent doctors in a number of clinics that used a binder system, and being unfamiliar with the patients, this was a huge issue because I had nothing to refer back to—I was essentially flying blind. I would see a new patient on the last day of a billing cycle, and when he would come back next visit, his initial exam would be gone. At best, this slows everything down if you have to go try to track down records during a visit, so you know what's going on with a patient.

I strongly advise against using the ring binder system—it's convenient, but it's a very bad way of keeping clinical records. If you're an employee, you may not have a choice, but in that case, I would suggest making a strong argument to your employer to change to a folder system. It's better for everyone's benefit and protection.

Content—SOAPs

Having a well-structured record system doesn't mean much if the recordkeeping itself is lacking. Clinical information and daily SOAP notes need to be recorded thoroughly. Having covered and worked in dozens of no-fault clinics, I've seen some good notes and recordkeeping, and I've seen plenty of bad.

When treatment is billed to no-fault insurance, the carrier has the right, by regulation, to request a report for that visit and for every visit or treatment billed. No-fault clinics will always send in the daily SOAPs for each visit along with the bills to avoid delays in payment from requests for missing notes.

No-fault billing is not like Medicare; it doesn't take much to satisfy the requirements to be reimbursed. (After all, most of Zemlyansky and company's claims were paid.) As long as the basic information is there (a complaint, findings, and a treatment) and the notes are signed, bills must be paid or denied within thirty days. As long as the treatment is supported by the diagnosis, and absent a specific reason for denial, bills are usually paid. Therefore, the detail level of many clinics' daily SOAP notes is designed basically to be just adequate to get paid.

In the SOAP sheet favored by many clinics I've worked in, there are spaces to check off areas of pain and perhaps pain level (S), areas of spasm, tenderness and subluxation (O), whether there has been improvement or not (A), and what adjustment and other procedures were performed (P). There are also spaces for both patient and chiropractor to sign. All this can be packed into a block not much bigger than this paragraph, with several more identical blocks on one page.

Of course, chiropractic visits are by nature repetitive, and very often not much varies visit to visit. Also, chiropractic visits in a no-fault clinic can reach numbers in the dozens, and having a system that is economical with paper is understandable. But many of these SOAP "blocks" leave little to no room for anything handwritten and do not take into account variability of subjective complaints in different areas. For example, a SOAP block may have check-off boxes for "pain" in C, T, and L areas. If a patient has both neck and low back pain on a given visit, you would check off C and L. But is the pain constant or intermittent? More frequent now or less than two weeks ago? What if the neck pain was mild and intermittent and the low back pain was constant and severe? What if the lower back had been mild but just got worse? What if the pain is on the left? What if it used to be on the right? What if the patient has a new complaint? There's often nowhere to write this but to try and cram it into a white space somewhere or in the margin. Not exactly ideal clinical recordkeeping.

The record should tell a story—the story of that patient's care, from beginning to present date. It should have enough information so that if it were picked up by someone unfamiliar with the case—like, say, a covering doctor—it would tell that doctor everything clinically necessary about that patient to seamlessly continue care.

No-fault clinics deal in high patient volume, so it's not unusual for a chiropractor to see 40, 50, or even 60 patients a day in a busy office. At peak times a chiropractor can see 10 patients an hour, with very little time to write detailed notes. Also, chiropractic treatment can be very repetitive; patients are coming in several times a week, and complaints, findings, and treatment will often not vary much by visit—but sometimes they do. The check-off blocks are okay for routine, uncomplicated visits, and often not much more is necessary. But sometimes the clinical situation changes, and there needs to be enough room to account for it adequately. There also needs to be a provision in the notes system for updating complaints and findings at regular intervals, be it a full re-examination or just an expanded SOAP. It's too easy to just keep checking off the same things every visit, and before you know it you have six pages and thirty visits that all say basically the same thing. Again, the record should tell a story—and that's not a story.

Daily SOAPs should also ideally indicate not only what areas were adjusted, but which technique was used and if there was any negative reaction. I've seen check-off forms where only the area of adjustment was listed (C, T, L), but there was nowhere to indicate how it was adjusted. Was it Diversified? Activator? Blocking? Flexion? Just soft-tissue work and mobilization? It matters, especially if the patient had increased pain after a visit, or if a cover doctor is seeing the patient.

The SOAP acronym, as we all know, denotes the patient's *S*ubjective complaints, the doctor's *O*bjective findings, the *A*ssessment of the patient's progress and condition at that visit, and the treatment *P*lan. The check-off area for complaints in the SOAP block may be adequate for most patients, for a routine visit. However, it's a good practice to use the patient's own words in the chief complaint whenever possible. For example, if a patient has daily complaints of lower back pain, and walks in one day and says, "My back's killin' me today, doc"—*write it in the patient's chart: Pt states "my back's killin' me today."* Yes, it takes three more seconds to write. But it conveys much more than just checking off an "L" under Complaints; it tells a story.

Content—Plan

As mentioned earlier, once the patient has been examined and given a diagnosis, a treatment plan is formulated and recorded in the file. This initial treatment plan should be tailored to the individual patient and should include visit frequency, technique, prognosis, goals, and a re-evaluation point. In many clinics, however, the initial examination report contains a brief, generic "plan" that reads something like:

"Patient will be treated 3-4 times a week with specific spinal manipulation to restore proper spinal function, alignment, and mobility, and will be re-evaluated in 4-6 weeks." I suggest adding a brief handwritten plan in the chart after the initial exam with something like the following:

Plan: light manual mobiliz C/S & L/S and/or L/S flexion to tolerance 1-2 wks while in acute pain, progressing to light Div CMT C/S & L/S if tolerated.

That's it—just a short note telling yourself, and any other chiropractor that might see the patient, what you plan to do. I've often gone to cover clinics where I'd never worked before, and been faced with patients coming in for the second time, who had their initial visit and examination with the other chiropractor. A note like this would have been extremely helpful.

On a daily visit basis, the "P"—plan will either be to continue with the initial plan or change it. If you originally began treating the patient with light technique or mobilization only because the patient was in too much pain to tolerate anything else, but has now improved, write for that visit that the patient has improved, that light Diversified was introduced to the areas you adjusted, and that it was tolerated well. Indicate that this will continue going forward.

We've all been taught what proper clinical recordkeeping is and how to do it. We've all heard the axiom, "if it wasn't written [in the chart], it wasn't done." And while no-fault clinics are busy places where chart space is economized, and patient visit time can be short, there's no reason why recordkeeping in a no-fault clinic should be *qualitatively* different from recordkeeping in a general chiropractic practice. If anything, chiropractic records should be more detailed. Writing short longhand notes where indicated, or at least every few visits is a good practice that helps tell the story of the patient's care and also protects you and the profession.

15

DISCHARGE

Discharge means releasing a patient from treatment once they have reached full or maximum recovery. Chiropractors are well-known for not discharging patients; we've been taught (mostly by chiropractic marketing and "practice-building" companies) to build lifetime relationships with them and to transition them to ongoing maintenance or wellness care. Many patients also have the notion that chiropractic care is something that "once you start, you have to keep going." I've heard this from more than one patient, and I'm sure that if you're reading this, you've heard it as well. There's even a popular joke about it:

Q: How many chiropractors does it take to change a light bulb?

A: Only one, but it takes thirty-six visits, three times a week.

Chiropractors weren't always averse to discharging patients. The aphorism "find it, fix it, and leave it alone" ("it" being the subluxation or spinal lesion), believed to be coined by the founder of osteopathic medicine, Andrew Taylor Still (1828-1917), was also adopted by early chiropractor Clarence Gonstead (1898-1978).[63] They believed that once the patient's problem had been corrected, the patient no longer needed care—in other words, they were discharged.

Wellness or maintenance care is not necessarily a bad thing, certainly not in chiropractic general practice. And, chronic conditions obviously need regular ongoing management as well. But no-fault insurance was never intended to provide wellness care or lifetime management of chronic conditions—it was intended to get patients better, advancing them towards a therapeutic goal. However, in most no-fault clinics where I have worked, patients are rarely discharged. Of course, many patients are still complaining of symptoms and/or have become chronic, and so they still need care; I'm not talking about them. But there are patients in no-fault clinics who have improved, who are no longer complaining of pain or other symptoms and have not in a while, and yet still come in for care. These patients may be a minority, but they do exist. There are generally two ways patients leave a no-fault practice: their treatment is ended after an IME by the insurance carrier, or they simply stop coming, usually because they feel better.

Around twelve weeks after the date of their accident, patients will typically receive a letter from their no-fault insurance carrier instructing them to report for an independent examination (known as an IME, or Independent Medical Examination, although the process applies to chiropractors and acupuncturists as well). These examinations are conducted by providers contracted with the

---

[63] The epigram, "Find the subluxations- correct it- leave it alone" is engraved on Gonstead's headstone in Mount Horeb Union Cemetery in Mt. Horeb, WI.

insurance carrier for that objective, usually through a middleman company. The purpose of the examination is to determine if the patient has reached *maximum medical improvement* (MMI). If the examiner determines that MMI has been reached, the carrier will no longer reimburse for further treatment, and the patient and all treating providers will be notified by letter of the determination and the effective date. After having their care (or the reimbursement for their care) ended following an IME, many patients simply stop coming.

Patients will often tell you when they have gotten a letter to go see "the insurance doctor". It's important to explain the nature of the IME to patients, and to explain to them that the IME doctor is not their advocate. Many patients misunderstand this, as we saw in Jessica's case in Chapter 13.

While the fairness of the IME *process* and industry is certainly up for discussion, the IME concept itself is not an unreasonable one. No-fault benefits were never intended to be indefinite. The goal of treatment is to return the patient to pre-injury status, or as close to it as possible. Continued treatment is reasonable as long as the treatment is effective and the patient continues to improve. When the patient reaches a plateau, and no further clinical benefit can be achieved, the insurance will not cover continued treatment that is not resulting in therapeutic progress.

Again, many patients have real injuries that can become chronic, and continue to have complaints of pain right up to their IMEs. They should not necessarily be discharged. There are avenues of recourse for these patients: care can be continued on a lien basis or can be continued and the bills for post-IME care settled through litigation or arbitration with the no-fault carrier. Or, patients can use commercial health insurance (such as Blue Cross) if they have it, as long as the IME denial is submitted with the claims. However, patients who consistently deny having pain or symptoms for several weeks, and who show objective signs of recovery—no spinal tenderness, full range of motion, no leg length difference, no subluxation, no abnormal provocative tests—should be released from care. There's no clinical reason not to.

Most dedicated no-fault clinics don't do this. Very often, it's because the clinic wants to keep generating revenue, and the lawyers and the clinic staff tell patients to keep coming—which they do. I have found that especially in busy clinics, it's easy to get into a routine of seeing patients on autopilot—the patient comes in, a brief greeting, maybe you ask, "how are you feeling?", you adjust them, and repeat with the next patient. But if you actually take a moment, sit down with a patient and directly ask about their symptoms in a detailed manner, you'll get more detailed answers. In other words, you have to re-evaluate the patient on a regular basis. If you only ask, "how are you feeling today?" you'll probably get answers like, "about the same," "a little better," or, "a lot of pain." Instead, regularly ask questions like:

- How is the pain in your (neck, back)?
- Are you having pain as frequently as you were a month ago?
- Are you generally feeling less pain now than when you first started care?
- When was the last time you had pain?
- Are you able to sleep better?
- Have you returned to work?

A good practice is to have the patient complete an outcome questionnaire like the Oswestry and Roland-Morris once a month. Some clinics actually do this already. (The questionnaires can be found in Appendix B of this book.)

Of course, before a patient is discharged, their visit frequency is usually tapered downward over their course of treatment, depending on the nature of their injuries and their progress. In no-fault clinics, most patients are typically prescribed an initial course of care at a frequency of 3-4 times per week for the first 4-6 weeks. This visit frequency usually applies to their physical therapy and acupuncture treatment as well as to their chiropractic care. As they improve, their visits should be reduced to 2-3 times per week for 4-6 weeks, and then to 1-2 visits per week for 4 weeks, or a similar sort of schedule.

As we have repeatedly discussed, the only way to know if a patient is improving is to regularly reassess their progress. Patients may be initially prescribed a visit frequency of 3-4 times per week for all their treatments, but often have injuries to different areas that may be improving at different rates, and so they may need chiropractic care at a greater or lesser frequency than physical therapy. An example that I've often encountered is when a patient has injuries to their spine and also has a torn knee meniscus and/or a rotator cuff. They are initially prescribed physical therapy, acupuncture, and chiropractic care 3-4 times per week for 4-6 weeks. After eight weeks of continued knee or shoulder pain, they may undergo arthroscopic surgical repair; they then need post-surgical physical therapy 3-4 times a week for 6 weeks. But their back pain may have improved within 4 or 6 weeks, and so now they may only need to be adjusted once or twice a week. Unless you have re-evaluated that patient for the necessity of continued chiropractic care, they may continue to present to you for adjustments because they have been conditioned to see you at the same rate as their other therapy. It's up to you as the treating chiropractor to set the *chiropractic* treatment schedule.

After the patient has been on a schedule of 1 visit per week for around 2-3 weeks, it is probably time to consider discharging the patient. If you're a chiropractor practicing in a dedicated no-fault clinic, you won't be able to completely discharge a patient from the facility. Unless you're their only provider, the patient is receiving other treatment under the care of the medical director, and only the medical director can make a determination for discharge from physical therapy and other medical care. (The same is true for acupuncturists and acupuncture.) But again, only you as the chiropractor can determine the necessity and appropriateness of chiropractic treatment.

If you determine that the patient no longer needs active, regular care, you can begin the discharge process. One way this can be done is with a "trial withdrawal" of care—a short period, say, two weeks—of no treatment. Then follow up with the patient to see if they have regressed or remained stable. If they have remained stable and symptom-free, with no objective findings, you can probably safely discharge them. If they have had some pain or symptoms in the interim, you can resume treatment at the frequency that was effective before.

If explicitly discharging patients is still something you're not comfortable with for some reason, I suggest that instead, you change their care plan to be seen "as needed," and place the patient on "PRN (L., *pro re nata*—'for an occasion that has arisen') status." I have done this after patients have come in denying pain for two or three weeks after months of care, and without objective findings. Tell the patient that while you cannot stop any of their other treatments, it appears that there is no chiropractic treatment needed today and to come back and see you only if pain returns. Of course, write the patient's new plan in the chart. If there are other chiropractors involved in the patient's care, it is important to discuss changing any plan with them and agree on any course of action.

There may not be many patients to discharge; often patients get sent to the IME process and leave care before they can be formally discharged. Personally, I believe that no-fault insurers are sending patients to IME earlier than they have in the past. Also, like many chiropractors, I believe that most patients need more care than the insurance companies and the IME examiners are willing to allow. But, some patients don't, and they just get better with the care we give them.

Imagine that! Patients getting better with chiropractic.

NO-FAULT WITH NO FEAR

16

WORKING FOR A LIVING

Congratulations! You've just graduated from chiropractic school. After almost four years of hard work, you're ready to go out and practice. Or, maybe you are already working in a practice, but are looking for a new opportunity; or perhaps you've just moved to a new area. Whatever the situation, you've got student loans, bills to pay, and possibly a family to support. Now you have to find work.

Unless you have tens of thousands of dollars in capital handy or the credit to get a business loan, and a strong business and marketing plan to build a practice, you'll need to find regular paid work. Even if you plan on starting your own practice, you might need to work part-time to pay the bills as you grow your practice. It's what I did when I began my private practice; I worked two or three days a week in no-fault clinics while seeing patients in my office and building my practice the rest of the week. And if you have to find paid work as a chiropractor, it's a fairly good bet that you'll be working in a no-fault clinic. As I showed in chapter 5 of this book, about half of available chiropractic employment opportunities are in no-fault.

As I also mentioned earlier in this book, it is very common in the New York metropolitan area for chiropractors to enter arrangements with several no-fault clinics and hire employee doctors to work in them. Mostly, the motivation is to make money; as long as there's a doctor—any doctor—to see the clinic's patients, visits can be billed, revenue generated, and overhead covered, hopefully with a profit for the employer. There's nothing wrong with that—it's a business, and the first goal of any business is to make money, otherwise, you can't stay in business. The problem is, as chiropractors we don't just sell widgets; we provide health care, and providing health care means we have a fiduciary duty to the patients. By the same token, being an employer means there are fiduciary responsibilities to the employee.

There seems to be a very high turnover rate for employee chiropractors in no-fault clinics. If you're a regular visitor to the most popular chiropractic career opportunities websites, over time you'll notice that some of the same employers are posting ads every couple of months or so.

Why is this so? Well, for one thing, no-fault work can be hard. As I mentioned earlier, many no-fault offices are in bad neighborhoods, with poor parking, and have long hours with high patient volumes. I've had many part-time jobs in such clinics, and have done coverage jobs in many others, and I couldn't envision working full-time in such places. Spending ten hours a day in a small, windowless room (sometimes in a basement), seeing 40, 50, or even 70 patients a day—some of whom do not speak much or any English—with a crappy torn adjusting table, the wrong size face paper, and an uncomfortable chair to sit on is not an appealing way to spend 50 hours a week. In fact, it's absolute drudgery. Not surprisingly, many chiropractors would rather not work full-time in such clinics. In fact, all things being equal, I would rather have two or three part-time jobs in different clinics rather than work full-time in one, just to break the monotony a little. And many chiropractors do just that, because it can be that depressing. Consequently, working chiropractors may be frequently switching part-time jobs until they find ones they can be more comfortable in—always keeping an ear to the ground for a better opportunity.

Also, offices frequently close, or change "ownership." More than once, I've worked for a chiropractor who just "took over the P.C." in a clinic. This meant the previous chiropractor left or was ousted by the clinic management for some reason. Either way, it meant that someone was unhappy, or worse, in some kind of trouble. I always took this as a dubious omen, and you should too, because it never worked out well for me. When a new chiropractor takes over and brings his P.C. into a clinic, it's usually as a business opportunity; they have several other similar clinics, and since they don't plan on seeing patients there themselves unless they have to, they hire an employee doc. I get the feeling that this kind of thing happens more than just occasionally, and that this contributes to the "associate ad churn" that appears on chiropractic employment job boards.

A word about patient volumes is warranted here. As mentioned in Chapter 2, patient volumes in no-fault clinics are usually high—around 40 chiropractic patients a day is typical, and around 60 is not unusual. However, I have worked in offices where the volume was as high as 90.

A comfortable daily patient volume is around 30. Doing routine adjustments only, and maybe a few stretches or demonstrating exercises, a reasonably experienced chiropractor can see about ten established patients in an hour, working at a brisk pace. In most offices that see typical volumes around 40-60 daily visits, that pace will exist for only the busier hours—usually in the afternoon, when the after-work patients come in. In offices where the volume reaches 70-90, the chiropractor will have to keep up that pace most of the day.

In my opinion, the number of patients one chiropractor sees per day in a no-fault setting should not exceed 50-60. I don't care what anyone tells you—seeing any more than that is unsustainable and will burn you out. More importantly, after 50 patients you will be fatigued, your technique will suffer, and it's just not good clinical practice. If you are working in a clinic where average daily patient visits reach 70-90 a day, you should probably start looking for a new place to work.

Whether you're a chiropractor who has an associate working in your clinic, or you're working for another doctor in his, there are some basic principles to keep in mind that will ensure that employers, employees, and patients all benefit.

If You Are an Employer

If you are a chiropractor who employs other chiropractors in your no-fault practice, below are some suggestions based on my experience being employed by chiropractors in dozens of no-fault clinics.

Pay Well. I've seen quite a few ads, even recently, for jobs offering $25 an hour. Doctors, it's not 1996 anymore. Yes, you need to make money, but so do we. Most clinics have ten-hour days, and $250 a day in the NYC area is just not adequate today. It's no secret how much a chiropractic visit bills out for under no-fault, and when we see 40 or more patients a day, we can do basic math. A minimum of $300 a day or $35 an hour is fair, and you can afford to pay an employee doctor a decent rate for a hard day's work. Don't skimp on pay, or you'll always be looking for new chiropractors. (And there's that "ad churn" again.)

Pay on Time. I've lost count of how many times I've worked for other chiropractors where checks have bounced, been late, and were miscalculated. I'm not talking about "honest" mistakes or forgetfulness. One doctor for whom I'd worked a week and a half coverage didn't pay me for months afterward, kept putting me off when I called and messaged him, and finally stopped answering my calls and e-mails. I finally had to confront him in person in his office, unannounced, where he asked if I was going to beat him up. (Obviously, I said no.) Another doctor for whom I covered regularly kept not leaving checks for me and paying me late, making me have to constantly call him about it. Yet another doctor missed the very first payroll, and I had to repeatedly call him and hear him make excuses about the direct deposit "not going through." When he finally did make a payment deposit, the amount wasn't right. I asked him for a stub and found that he had miscalculated the taxes. I decided to cut my losses and quit after a month.

Playing games with payroll reflects poorly on you, both as an employer and as a professional. It causes your employees untold aggravation, having to hound you constantly and feel like *they're* the jerk for doing it. They have bills of their own to pay. Not paying on time is also a sign that a business is doing poorly. If you are having "cash flow problems," you still need to figure out how to pay your employees on time, because if you don't, they *will* quit.

Provide Decent Equipment. Nothing says, "I don't really give a damn about my patients/employees/office" like a cramped room, a tiny desk and chair, and a bench table with no movable headpiece and torn upholstery. Aesthetically, the implications are obvious. If you went to a dentist, what would you think if you saw an old decrepit dental chair with torn vinyl and leaking stuffing? Is it possible to adjust patients on a torn-up bench table? Sure it is. Can you provide better care on a table with more functionality? And does that reflect better upon you and the employees you hire, and on chiropractic in general? Yes, yes, and yes.

Of course, as I've said earlier, some chiropractors see an opportunity to "bring their P.C." to a no-fault clinic as just another turn-key, money-making venture; the patients are already there, so just plug in a chiropractor and go, and who needs fancy equipment. I'm not talking fancy—I'm talking decent. If you want patients to *want* to receive chiropractic care in your no-fault practice, start by making it a little more appealing—or at least not *unappealing*. Trust me, it goes a long way.

Let Your Doctors be Doctors. The chiropractor treating the patient must make the clinical decisions; if more than one chiropractor is regularly seeing a patient, they should communicate with each other regarding any clinical issues or differences in approach. More than that, though, the treating doctor(s) should not be pressured to order tests, imaging, or durable medical equipment, and should have the freedom to change a patient's visit frequency or discharge a patient. Even if you're the doctor signing the checks, the treating doctor's name should be in block 16 of the NF-3 form (see Appendix C)—and he or she should be the one making clinical decisions.

Use Proper Employment Structure. Many employer chiropractors pay their associates or cover doctors as independent contractors, or "on a 1099." This might be easier for the employer because the employee has to pay their own taxes, there's no Worker's Compensation insurance necessary (depending on the number of hours), and the bookkeeping is easier. However, it's also against New York State Insurance Law and your bills might not be paid if the services were actually rendered by a doctor who was paid as an independent contractor (IC).

From the NYS Department of Financial Services website:

> "(a) Where the owner(s) of a PC is licensed to perform health services and such service are performed by a PC owner or an employee under the supervision of a PC owner, the services may be billed for under No-Fault by the PC as the licensed provider of those services.
>
> (b) Where the health services are performed by a provider who is an independent contractor with the PC and is not an employee under the direct supervision of a PC owner, the PC is not authorized to bill under No-Fault as a licensed provider of those services.
>
> ...since the control, and therefore the liability, of the principal for the acts of the independent contractor is attenuated, and in order to preserve the integrity of the No-Fault and physician licensing systems, this Department has determined that, when the services are provided by an independent contractor, the PC should not be considered as the "licensed provider" authorized to bill under No-Fault."

Paying your employee doctors as ICs may result in your bills not being paid, or worse, having to be paid back, if a no-fault insurer discovers that the services it paid for were improperly rendered by an IC. (Of course, you could lie, and put your own name in block 16 of the NF-3, but I would advise against that.) One doctor for whom I did frequent per diem coverage work told me, when I first began working for him, to not sign my SOAP notes. In fact, he was quite annoyed with me when he saw that I had. The reason, I quickly figured out, was because he was paying me as an IC, and if I signed my SOAPs—which were sent to the insurer along with the bills—there would be other signatures than his, raising the question of whose they were and the nature of the employment relationship, and jeopardizing his reimbursement. I informed him that there was no way I would not be signing my SOAP notes and that I was happy to be paid as a W-2 employee instead of an IC. (Putting aside the myriad other legal and ethical problems raised by him signing someone else's treatment notes.)

If you're the employer chiropractor, it's worthwhile to "play by the book" in this regard. Yes, it takes a bit more time to set up with a payroll company, especially if you frequently hire different cover doctors, and might cost a little bit extra in Comp insurance. But as the employer and P.C. owner, you're carrying all the risk here—pay a cover doc as an IC and he still gets paid, but you still have to worry about the carrier deciding to ask you for repayment for services improperly rendered by an IC.

(See http://www.dfs.ny.gov/insurance/ogco2001/rg102212.htm)

If You Are an Employee

Whether you're a full-time associate doctor, a part-time doc or just covering a no-fault practice for a day or a week, there are some important things to keep in mind (and many of these apply to employers, too):

Be on Time. This is good advice no matter what job you have or profession you're in. No one likes to be kept waiting. Showing up late reflects poorly on you and on chiropractic.

Interact Well with the Staff and Patients. This may seem obvious, but you'd be surprised. Staff are often overworked, and patients are often in pain. If you're a cover doctor, you're another new face and patients might be apprehensive of how you're going to be treating them. A professional and personable demeanor and a good bedside manner make people more comfortable with you, and are therapeutically beneficial as well.

Get Paid. If you're full-time and on a regular W-2 payroll, you hopefully will not need to worry about this much. But if you're working several part-time jobs, or doing a lot of coverage work in different offices every week for new employers, make sure you get paid and on time. It won't happen often, but it will happen that an employer will be late with a check. If it happens more than once within a period of time, you may want to consider whether your employer has a healthy operation. If you are covering for a doctor for the first time, or in a clinic where you haven't worked before, it's always a good idea to ask for a check to be waiting for you at the office, and let the hiring doctor know that this is your policy before you accept the job. If you will be covering more than one day, ask that it be post-dated the last day of coverage. You don't want to have to chase people for your money.

Ask to be paid on a W-2; you won't have to worry about paying estimated quarterly taxes, and as was mentioned earlier, no-fault treatment services rendered as an IC are ineligible for reimbursement. Again, that is more of an issue for the employer than for the employee, but it is best to play by the book.

Be the Doctor. To paraphrase the title of a book authored by an icon of the chiropractic profession, the late Dr. Fred Barge (1933-2003), you are the doctor, doctor. You make the chiropractic clinical decisions for the patients that you see—not the staff, not the clinic managers, and not even the doctor you work for who has never seen the patient. If you think an MRI or a lumbar brace is necessary, order one. If you don't think so, don't—and stand by your decision. (Document it too, of course.) Your first duty is to what is in the best interest of the patient, not the employer, and if your job is threatened because of it, then you probably shouldn't be working there anyway.

Don't Get Caught up in the Numbers Game. Some employers and clinic staff are very concerned with the number of patients seen by the chiropractor; they often collect the sign-in sheets from the different providers and compare the numbers of patients seen. Every patient seen is viewed as money in the bank, and patients not seen are money left on the table. A complaint often heard by employee doctors is that they haven't seen nearly as many patients as physical therapy. The reasoning is that since most patients are receiving both chiropractic and physical therapy, the numbers of patients seen by the two disciplines should be very close.

Of course, this reasoning is obviously flawed; patients may get physical therapy but not chiropractic for a variety of reasons. Sometimes their injuries are too acute, and they are not yet ready. Sometimes they have clinical contraindications (spinal hardware, etc.) They may need physical therapy for their knee three times a week, but chiropractic only once a week. They may be in a rush, and not want to wait. Or, they may just not want to receive chiropractic care for other reasons.

My advice? Don't sweat it. Of course, a practice is a business, as we've said before, and businesses must make money. By all means, be conscientious, work hard, and see patients efficiently at a pace you are comfortable with. But patients should already know that you are there and that they should be seeing you, and it's not your job to chase after them if they want to leave. You're the doctor; worry about the patients waiting for you, not the ones who decide they don't need you.

Whether you are the owner of a clinic practice, or you are a working associate chiropractor or itinerant coverage doctor, the best advice is to always follow the "No Fear" Principles:

Know who you are working for and with. Don't let anyone dictate how or how often you treat patients. Don't be a straw owner or become involved with them or other illegitimate business arrangements. Treat patients the way you would want a family member to be treated—objectively, and with clinical goals foremost in mind rather than financial interests or quotas. Document extensively, and be meticulous in your charting. Everything else will take care of itself.

AFTERWORD

I wrote this book because I love the chiropractic profession. Like probably many of you, I didn't plan to spend most of my career treating motor vehicle accident injuries, but I did, and I'd like to think that I got fairly good at it. But I also got frustrated at the industry, and some of the people in it—including other chiropractors—for treating the no-fault system as just another means to make a buck. I got frustrated at feeling like an instrument—just a cog in a big machine whose purpose was only to churn through as many patient visits as possible and make money for greedy clinic owners, lawyers, and the chiropractors I was working for. I was saddened and dismayed when I would see no-fault fraud reported in the news, and even more saddened when I would see chiropractors named as defendants. I worked in some lousy clinics, for some lousy doctors, and unfortunately, I sometimes saw carelessness and uncaring in many of the clinics where I worked—towards patients, towards recordkeeping, and towards employees, myself included.

I also saw good things, and met so many interesting and wonderful patients. (I could have written a whole other book about them—and perhaps someday I will—but this book was not intended to be a memoir.) I met simple, yet complex, good people who just wanted to get better. I got to be a part of their care, helping them during a painful and stressful time and sometimes making a real difference in their lives. There was Jessica, who we met in Chapter 13. There was also the 89-year-old gentleman whose cervical x-rays I took and saw popcorn calcifications in both his carotids, occluding them 90-95% (he ultimately had endarterectomies, and his cardiologist said the accident probably saved his life because without it he would never have had x-rays). And there was everyone who sat up after an adjustment and said, "Wow—that feels better!"

It's easy to get discouraged working in an industry that has a reputation for being "the bottom of the healthcare barrel" and associated with "ambulance chasers." But like so much else in life, it's all about attitude; I've always felt that by taking pride in yourself and in your profession, and by being unimpeachably ethical and acting with the highest degree of professionalism, you can rise above your surroundings. Of course, vigilance and propriety are paramount, and distancing yourself from illegal and potentially illegal activity is vital. But there's honest work out there; we just have to do it honestly, and with integrity. I wanted to do something to improve things in some small way, and I hope that by writing this book, I have accomplished that.

We still have a ways to go, of course; self-improvement is a never-ending process, be it at the personal level, as professionals, or across an entire industry. But I hope that the information I have presented in the preceding pages will be a beginning, and a continuation, of a journey we are all of us on together.

"Out there in those great open spaces are multitudes seeking what you possess. The burdens are heavy; responsibilities are many; obligations are providential; but the satisfaction of traveling the populated highways and byways, relieving suffering and adding millions of years to lives of millions of suffering people, will bring forth satisfaction and glories with greater blessings than you think. Time is of the essence...for you have in your possession a sacred trust. Guard it well."

—From B.J. Palmer's last printed words

NO-FAULT WITH NO FEAR

APPENDIX A

Article 51 of the New York Insurance Law aka "The No-Fault Law"

5101. Title.

This article shall be known and may be cited as the "Comprehensive Motor Vehicle Insurance Reparations Act."

5102. Definitions. In this chapter:

(a) "Basic economic loss" means, up to fifty thousand dollars per person of the following combined items, subject to the limitations of section five thousand one hundred eight of this article:

(1) All necessary expenses incurred for:

(i) medical, hospital (including services rendered in compliance with article forty-one of the public health law, whether or not such services are rendered directly by a hospital), surgical, nursing, dental, ambulance, x-ray, prescription drug and prosthetic services;

(ii) psychiatric, physical and occupational therapy and rehabilitation*;

NOTE: Section 5102(a)(1)(ii) of the New York Insurance Law has been amended, effective November 23, 2006, to read as follows:

(ii) psychiatric, physical therapy (provided that treatment is rendered pursuant to a referral) and occupational therapy and rehabilitation;

(iii) any non-medical remedial care and treatment rendered in accordance with a religious method of healing recognized by the laws of this state; and

(iv) any other professional health services; all without limitation as to time, provided that within one year after the date of the accident causing the injury it is ascertainable that further expenses may be incurred as a result of the injury. For the purpose of determining basic economic loss, the expenses incurred under this paragraph shall be in accordance with the limitations of section five thousand one hundred eight of this article.

(2) Loss of earnings from work which the person would have performed had he not been injured, and reasonable and necessary expenses incurred by such person in obtaining services in lieu of those that he would have performed for income, up to two thousand dollars per month for not more than three years from the date of the accident causing the injury. An employee who is entitled to receive monetary payments, pursuant to statute or contract with the employer, or who receives voluntary monetary benefits paid for by the employer, by reason of the employee's inability to work because of personal injury arising out of the use or operation of a motor vehicle, is not entitled to receive first party benefits for "loss of earnings from work" to the extent that such monetary payments or benefits from the employer do not result in the employee suffering a reduction in income or a reduction in the employee's level of future benefits arising from a subsequent illness or injury.

(3) All other reasonable and necessary expenses incurred, up to twenty-five dollars per day for not more than one year from the date of the accident causing the injury.

(4) "Basic economic loss" shall not include any loss incurred on account of death; subject, however, to the provisions of paragraph four of subsection (a) of section five thousand one hundred three of this article.

(5) "Basic economic loss" shall also include an additional option to purchase, for an additional premium, an additional twenty-five thousand dollars of coverage which the insured or his legal representative may specify will be applied to loss of earnings from work and/or psychiatric, physical or occupational therapy and rehabilitation after the initial fifty thousand dollars of basic economic loss has been exhausted. This optional additional

coverage shall be made available and notice with explanation of such coverage shall be provided by an insurer at the first policy renewal after the effective date of this paragraph, or at the time of application.

(b) "First party benefits" means payments to reimburse a person for basic economic loss on account of personal injury arising out of the use or operation of a motor vehicle, less:

(1) Twenty percent of lost earnings computed pursuant to paragraph two of subsection (a) of this section.

(2) Amounts recovered or recoverable on account of such injury under state or federal laws providing social security disability benefits, or workers' compensation benefits, or disability benefits under article nine of the workers' compensation law, or Medicare benefits, other than lifetime reserve days and provided further that the Medicare benefits utilized herein do not result in a reduction of such person's Medicare benefits for a subsequent illness or injury.

(3) Amounts deductible under the applicable insurance policy.

(c) "Non-economic loss" means pain and suffering and similar non-monetary detriment.

(d) "Serious injury" means a personal injury which results in death; dismemberment; significant disfigurement; a fracture; loss of a fetus; permanent loss of use of a body organ, member, function or system; permanent consequential limitation of use of a body organ or member; significant limitation of use of a body function or system; or a medically determined injury or impairment of a non-permanent nature which prevents the injured person from performing substantially all of the material acts which constitute such person's usual and customary daily activities for not less than ninety days during the one hundred eighty days immediately following the occurrence of the injury or impairment.

(e) "Owner" means an owner as defined in section one hundred twenty-eight of the vehicle and traffic law.

(f) "Motor vehicle" means a motor vehicle as defined in section three hundred eleven of the vehicle and traffic law and also includes fire and police vehicles. It shall not include any motor vehicle not required to carry financial security pursuant to article six, eight or forty-eight-A of the vehicle and traffic law or a motorcycle, as defined in subsection (m) hereof.

(g) "Insurer" means the insurance company or self-insurer, as the case may be, which provides the financial security required by article six or eight of the vehicle and traffic law.

(h) "Member of his household" means a spouse, child or relative of the named insured who regularly resides in his household.

(i) "Uninsured motor vehicle" means a motor vehicle, the owner of which is (i) a financially irresponsible motorist as defined in subsection (j) of section five thousand two hundred two of this chapter or (ii) unknown and whose identity is unascertainable.

(j) "Covered person" means any pedestrian injured through the use or operation of, or any owner, operator or occupant of, a motor vehicle which has in effect the financial security required by article six or eight of the vehicle and traffic law or which is referred to in subdivision two of section three hundred twenty-one of such law; or any other person entitled to first party benefits.

(k) "Bus" means both a bus and a school bus as defined in sections one hundred four and one hundred forty-two of the vehicle and traffic law.

(l) "Compensation provider" means the state insurance fund, or the person, association, corporation or insurance carrier or statutory fund liable under state or federal laws for the payment of workers' compensation benefits or disability benefits under article nine of the workers' compensation law.

(m) "Motorcycle" means any motorcycle, as defined in section one hundred twenty-three of the vehicle and traffic law, and which is required to carry financial security pursuant to article six, eight or forty-eight-A of the vehicle and traffic law.

5103. Entitlement to first party benefits; additional financial security required.

(a) Every owner's policy of liability insurance issued on a motor vehicle in satisfaction of the requirements of article six or eight of the vehicle and traffic law shall also provide for; every owner who maintains another form of financial security on a motor vehicle in satisfaction of the requirements of such articles shall be liable for; and every owner of a motor vehicle required to be subject to the provisions of this article by subdivision two of section three hundred twenty-one of the vehicle and traffic law shall be liable for; the payment of first party benefits to:

(1) Persons, other than occupants of another motor vehicle or a motorcycle, for loss arising out of the use or operation in this state of such motor vehicle. In the case of occupants of a bus other than operators, owners, and employees of the owner or operator of the bus, the coverage for first party benefits shall be afforded under the policy or policies, if any, providing first party benefits to the injured person and members of his household for loss arising out of the use or operation of any motor vehicle of such household. In the event there is no such policy, first party benefits shall be provided by the insurer of such bus.

(2) The named insured and members of his household, other than occupants of a motorcycle, for loss arising out of the use or operation of (i) an uninsured motor vehicle or motorcycle, within the United States, its territories or possessions, or Canada; and (ii) an insured motor vehicle or motorcycle outside of this state and within the United States, its territories or possessions, or Canada.

(3) Any New York resident who is neither the owner of a motor vehicle with respect to which coverage for first party benefits is required by this article nor, as a member of a household, is entitled to first party benefits under paragraph two of this subsection, for loss arising out of the use or operation of the insured or self-insured motor vehicle outside of this state and within the United States, its territories or possessions, or Canada.

(4) The estate of any covered person, other than an occupant of another motor vehicle or a motorcycle, a death benefit in the amount of two thousand dollars for the death of such person arising out of the use or operation of such motor vehicle which is in addition to any first party benefits for basic economic loss.

(b) An insurer may exclude from coverage required by subsection (a) hereof a person who:

(1) Intentionally causes his own injury.

(2) Is injured as a result of operating a motor vehicle while in an intoxicated condition or while his ability to operate such vehicle is impaired by the use of a drug within the meaning of section eleven hundred ninety-two of the vehicle and traffic law.

(3) Is injured while he is:

(i) committing an act which would constitute a felony, or seeking to avoid lawful apprehension or arrest by a law enforcement officer, or

(ii) operating a motor vehicle in a race or speed test, or

(iii) operating or occupying a motor vehicle known to him to be stolen, or

(iv) operating or occupying any motor vehicle owned by such injured person with respect to which the coverage required by subsection (a) hereof is not in effect, or

(v) a pedestrian, through being struck by any motor vehicle owned by such injured pedestrian with respect to which the coverage required by subsection (a) hereof is not in effect, or

(vi) repairing, servicing or otherwise maintaining a motor vehicle if such conduct is within the course of a business of repairing, servicing or otherwise maintaining a motor vehicle and the injury occurs on the business premises.

(c) Insurance offered by any company to satisfy the requirements of subsection (a) hereof shall be offered (i) without a deductible and (ii) with a family deductible of up to two hundred dollars (which deductible shall apply only to the loss of the named insured and members of his household). The superintendent may approve a higher deductible in the case of insurance policies providing additional benefits or pursuant to a plan designed and implemented to coordinate first party benefits with other benefits.

(d) Insurance policy forms for insurance to satisfy the requirements of subsection (a) hereof shall be subject to approval pursuant to article twenty-three of this chapter. Minimum benefit standards for such policies and for self-insurers, and rights of subrogation, examination and other such matters, shall be established by regulation pursuant to section three hundred one of this chapter.

(e) Every owner's policy of liability insurance issued in satisfaction of article six or eight of the vehicle and traffic law shall also provide, when a motor vehicle covered by such policy is used or operated in any other state or in any Canadian province, insurance coverage for such motor vehicle at least in the minimum amount required by the laws of that state or province.

(f) Every owner's policy of liability insurance issued on a motorcycle or an all terrain vehicle in satisfaction of the requirements of article six or eight of the vehicle and traffic law or section twenty-four hundred seven of such law shall also provide for; every owner who maintains another form of financial security on a motorcycle or an all terrain vehicle in satisfaction of the requirements of such articles or section shall be liable for; and every owner of a motorcycle or an all terrain vehicle required to be subject to the provisions of this article by subdivision two of section three hundred twenty-one of such law shall be liable for; the payment of first party benefits to persons, other than the occupants of such motorcycle or all terrain vehicle, another motorcycle or all terrain vehicle, or any motor vehicle, for loss arising out of the use or operation of the motorcycle or all terrain vehicle within this state. Every insurer and self-insurer may exclude from the coverage required by this subsection a person who intentionally causes his own injury or is injured while committing an act which would constitute a felony or while seeking to avoid lawful apprehension or arrest by a law enforcement officer.

(g) A company authorized to provide the insurance specified in paragraph three of subsection (a) of section one thousand one hundred thirteen of this chapter or a corporation organized pursuant to article forty-three of this chapter may, individually or jointly, with the approval of the superintendent upon a showing that the company or corporation is qualified to provide for all of the items of basic economic loss specified in paragraph one of subsection (a) of section five thousand one hundred two of this article, provide coverage for such items of basic economic loss to the extent that an insurer would be required to provide under this article. Where a policyholder elects to be covered under such an arrangement the insurer providing coverage for the automobile shall be furnished with the names of all persons covered by the company or corporation under the arrangement and such persons shall not be entitled to benefits for any of the items of basic economic loss specified in such paragraph. The premium for the automobile insurance policy shall be appropriately reduced to reflect the elimination of coverage for such items of basic economic loss. Coverage by the automobile insurer of such eliminated items shall be effected or restored upon request by the insured and payment of the premium for such coverage. All companies and corporations providing coverage for items of basic economic loss pursuant to the authorization of this subsection shall have only those rights and obligations which are applicable to an insurer subject to this article.

(h) Any policy of insurance obtained to satisfy the financial security requirements of article six or eight of the vehicle and traffic law which does not contain provisions complying with the requirements of this article, shall be construed as if such provisions were embodied therein.

5104. Causes of action for personal injury.

(a) Notwithstanding any other law, in any action by or on behalf of a covered person against another covered person for personal injuries arising out of negligence in the use or operation of a motor vehicle in this state, there shall be no right of recovery for non-economic loss, except in the case of a serious injury, or for basic economic loss. The owner, operator or occupant of a motorcycle which has in effect the financial security required by article six or eight of the vehicle and traffic law, or which is referred to in subdivision two of section three hundred twenty-one of such law, shall not be subject to an action by or on behalf of a covered person for recovery for non-economic loss, except in the case of a serious injury, or for basic economic loss.

(b) In any action by or on behalf of a covered person, against a non—covered person, where damages for personal injuries arising out of the use or operation of a motor vehicle or a motorcycle may be recovered, an insurer which paid or is liable for first party benefits on account of such injuries has a lien against any recovery to the extent of benefits paid or payable by it to the covered person. No such action may be compromised by the covered person except with the written consent of the insurer, or with the approval of the court, or where the amount of such settlement exceeds fifty thousand dollars. The failure of such person to commence such action within two years after accrual gives the insurer a cause of action for the amount of first party benefits paid or payable against any person who may be liable to the covered person for his personal injuries. The insurer's cause of action shall be in addition to the cause of action of the covered person except that in any action subsequently commenced by the covered person for such injuries, the amount of his basic economic loss shall not be recoverable.

(c) Where there is no right of recovery for basic economic loss, such loss may nevertheless be pleaded and proved to the extent that it is relevant to the proof of non-economic loss.

5105. Settlement between insurers.

(a) Any insurer liable for the payment of first party benefits to or on behalf of a covered person and any compensation provider paying benefits in lieu of first party benefits which another insurer would otherwise be obligated to pay pursuant to subsection (a) of section five thousand one hundred three of this article or section five thousand two hundred twenty-one of this chapter has the right to recover the amount paid from the insurer of any other covered person to the extent that such other covered person would have been liable, but for the provisions of this article, to pay damages in an action at law. In any case, the right to recover exists only if at least one of the motor vehicles involved is a motor vehicle weighing more than six thousand five hundred pounds unloaded or is a motor vehicle used principally for the transportation of persons or property for hire. However, in the case of occupants of a bus other than operators, owners, and employees of the owner or operator of the bus, an insurer which, pursuant to paragraph one of subsection (a) of section five thousand one hundred three of this article, provides coverage for first party benefits for such occupants under a policy providing first party benefits to the injured person and members of his household for loss arising out of the use or operation of any vehicle of such household, shall have no right to recover the amount of such benefits from the insurer of such bus.

(b) The sole remedy of any insurer or compensation provider to recover on a claim arising pursuant to subsection (a) hereof, shall be the submission of the controversy to mandatory arbitration pursuant to procedures promulgated or approved by the superintendent. Such procedures shall also be utilized to resolve all disputes arising between insurers concerning their responsibility for the payment of first party benefits.

(c) The liability of an insurer imposed by this section shall not affect or diminish its obligations under any policy of bodily injury liability insurance.

5106. Fair claims settlement.

(a) Payments of first party benefits and additional first party benefits shall be made as the loss is incurred. Such benefits are overdue if not paid within thirty days after the claimant supplies proof of the fact and amount of loss sustained. If proof is not supplied as to the entire claim, the amount which is supported by proof is overdue if not paid within thirty days after such proof is supplied. All overdue payments shall bear interest at the rate of two percent per month. If a valid claim or portion was overdue, the claimant shall also be entitled to recover his attorney's reasonable fee, for services necessarily performed in connection with securing payment of the overdue claim, subject to limitations promulgated by the superintendent in regulations.

(b) Every insurer shall provide a claimant with the option of submitting any dispute involving the insurer's liability to pay first party benefits, or additional first party benefits, the amount thereof or any other matter which may arise pursuant to subsection (a) hereof to arbitration pursuant to simplified procedures to be promulgated or approved by the superintendent.

(c) An award by an arbitrator shall be binding except where vacated or modified by a master arbitrator in accordance with simplified procedures to be promulgated or approved by the superintendent. The grounds for vacating or modifying an arbitrator's award by a master arbitrator shall not be limited to those grounds for review set forth in article seventy-five of the civil practice law and rules. The award of a master arbitrator shall be binding except for the grounds for review set forth in article seventy-five of the civil practice law and rules, and provided further that where the amount of such master arbitrator's award is five thousand dollars or greater, exclusive of interest and attorney's fees, the insurer or the claimant may institute a court action to adjudicate the dispute de novo.

5107. Coverage for non-resident motorists.

(a) Every insurer authorized to transact or transacting business in this state, or controlling or controlled by or under common control by or with such an insurer, which sells a policy providing motor vehicle liability insurance coverage or any similar coverage in any state or Canadian province, shall include in each such policy coverage to satisfy the financial security requirements of article six or eight of the vehicle and traffic law and to provide for the payment of first party benefits pursuant to subsection (a) of section five thousand one hundred three of this article when a motor vehicle covered by such policy is used or operated in this state.

(b) Every policy described in subsection (a) hereof shall be construed as having the coverage required by subsection (a) of section five thousand one hundred three of this article.

5108. Limit on charges by providers of health services.

(a) The charges for services specified in paragraph one of subsection (a) of section five thousand one hundred two of this article and any further health service charges which are incurred as a result of the injury and which are in excess of basic economic loss, shall not exceed the charges permissible under the schedules prepared and established by the chairman of the workers' compensation board for industrial accidents, except where the insurer or arbitrator determines that unusual procedures or unique circumstances justify the excess charge.

(b) The superintendent, after consulting with the chairman of the workers' compensation board and the commissioner of health, shall promulgate rules and regulations implementing and coordinating the provisions of this article and the workers' compensation law with respect to charges for the professional health services specified in paragraph one of subsection (a) of section five thousand one hundred two of this article, including the establishment of schedules for all such services for which schedules have not been prepared and established by the chairman of the workers' compensation board.

(c) No provider of health services specified in paragraph one of subsection (a) of section five thousand one hundred two of this article may demand or request any payment in addition to the charges authorized pursuant to this section. Every insurer shall report to the commissioner of health any patterns of overcharging, excessive treatment or other improper actions by a health provider within thirty days after such insurer has knowledge of such pattern.

5109. Unauthorized providers of health services.

(a) The superintendent, in consultation with the commissioner of health and the commissioner of education, shall by regulation, promulgate standards and procedures for investigating and suspending or removing the authorization for providers of health services to demand or request payment for health services as specified in paragraph one of subsection (a) of section five thousand one hundred two of this article upon findings reached after investigation pursuant to this section. Such regulations shall ensure the same or greater due process provisions, including notice and opportunity to be heard, as those afforded physicians investigated under article two of the workers' compensation law and shall include provision for notice to all providers of health services of the provisions of this section and regulations promulgated thereunder at least ninety days in advance of the effective date of such regulations.

(b) The commissioner of health and the commissioner of education shall provide a list of the names of all providers of health services who the commissioner of health and the commissioner of education shall deem, after reasonable investigation, not authorized to demand or request any payment for medical services in connection with any claim under this article because such provider of health services:

(1) has been guilty of professional or other misconduct or incompetency in connection with medical services rendered under this article; or

(2) has exceeded the limits of his or her professional competence in rendering medical care under this article or has knowingly made a false statement or representation as to a material fact in any medical report made in connection with any claim under this article; or

(3) solicited, or has employed another to solicit for himself or herself or for another, professional treatment, examination or care of an injured person in connection with any claim under this article; or

(4) has refused to appear before, or to answer upon request of, the commissioner of health, the superintendent, or any duly authorized officer of the state, any legal question, or to produce any relevant information concerning his or her conduct in connection with rendering medical services under this article; or

(5) has engaged in patterns of billing for services which were not provided.

(c) Providers of health services shall refrain from subsequently treating for remuneration, as a private patient, any person seeking medical treatment under this article if such provider pursuant to this section has been prohibited from demanding or requesting any payment for medical services under this article. An injured claimant so treated or examined may raise this as a defense in any action by such provider for payment for treatment rendered at any time after such provider has been prohibited from demanding or requesting payment for medical services in connection with any claim under this article.

(d) The commissioner of health and the commissioner of education shall maintain and regularly update a database containing a list of providers of health services prohibited by this section from demanding or requesting any payment for health services connected to a claim under this article and shall make such information available to the public by means of a website and by a toll free number.

(e) Nothing in this section shall be construed as limiting in any respect the powers and duties of the commissioner of health, commissioner of education or the superintendent to investigate instances of misconduct by a health care provider and, after a hearing and upon written notice to the provider, to temporarily prohibit a provider of health services under such investigation from demanding or requesting any payment for medical services under this article for up to ninety days from the date of such notice.

NO-FAULT WITH NO FEAR

APPENDIX B—Clinical Forms

<u>Informed Consent for Chiropractic Spinal Manipulation and Treatment</u>

I hereby request and consent to the performance of chiropractic adjustments and other chiropractic procedures on myself (or on the patient named below for whom I am legally responsible) by the licensed doctors of chiropractic of this office or any doctor, who now or in the future, works as a relief doctor. I have had the opportunity to discuss with my chiropractic doctor the nature and purpose of chiropractic adjustments and other procedures and understand that spinal manipulation involves the doctor placing his or her hands or an instrument on my spine and delivering a quick thrust or impulse to the involved area(s). I also understand and am informed that, as in the practice of medicine, in the practice of chiropractic there are some risks to treatment including, but not limited to: fractures, disc injuries, strokes, dislocations, sprains, and soreness. These risks are extremely low. I further understand that there are risks of not receiving chiropractic treatment, such as non-improvement or worsening of condition, and that there alternatives to chiropractic treatment such as medical care and/or physical therapy. I understand and comprehend all such risks and complications. I do not expect the doctor to be able to anticipate and explain all risks and complications, and I wish to rely on the doctor to exercise judgment during the course of the procedure which the doctor feels at the time, based upon the facts then known, is in my best interest. I, by my signature below, confirm and accept care and therefore consent to and agree to those treatments deemed necessary by my chiropractic doctor to be in my best interest.

I have been informed and understand how my Patient Health Information will be used and I agree to these policies and procedures. I have also read, or have had read to me the above informed consent, authorization and release. I have had an opportunity to ask any and all questions about its content, and by signing below, I agree to the above-named procedures. I intend this consent form to cover the entire course of treatment for my present condition and for future condition(s) for which I seek treatment in this office.

Patient Signature: _____ Date: ____/____/_____

PrintedName:_____

Consent to Treatment of a Minor

I, being the parent or legal guardian of _____, a minor, give consent for any licensed chiropractor in this office to render treatment to the above.

_____

Signature of parent/guardian   Date

Oswestry Disability Questionnaire

This questionnaire has been designed to give us information as to how your **back or leg pain** is affecting your ability to manage in everyday life. Please answer by checking **one box in each section** for the statement which best applies to you. We realize you may consider that two or more statements in any one section apply, but please just shade out the spot that indicates the statement which **most clearly describes your problem**.

Section 1: Pain Intensity
- I have no pain at the moment
- The pain is very mild at the moment
- The pain is moderate at the moment
- The pain is fairly severe at the moment
- The pain is very severe at the moment
- The pain is the worst imaginable at the moment

Section 2: Personal Care (eg. washing, dressing)
- I can look after myself normally without causing extra pain
- I can look after myself normally but it causes extra pain
- It is painful to look after myself and I am slow and careful
- I need some help but can manage most of my personal care
- I need help every day in most aspects of self-care
- I do not get dressed, wash with difficulty and stay in bed

Section 3: Lifting
- I can lift heavy weights without extra pain
- I can lift heavy weights but it gives me extra pain
- Pain prevents me lifting heavy weights off the floor but I can manage if they are conveniently placed (eg. on a table)
- Pain prevents me lifting heavy weights but I can manage light to medium weights if they are conveniently positioned
- I can only lift very light weights
- I cannot lift or carry anything

Section 4: Walking*
- Pain does not prevent me walking any distance
- Pain prevents me from walking more than 1 mile
- Pain prevents me from walking more than ½ mile
- Pain prevents me from walking more than 100 yards
- I can only walk using a stick or crutches
- I am in bed most of the time

Section 5: Sitting
- I can sit in any chair as long as I like
- I can only sit in my favorite chair as long as I like
- Pain prevents me sitting more than one hour
- Pain prevents me from sitting more than 30 minutes
- Pain prevents me from sitting more than 10 minutes
- Pain prevents me from sitting at all

Section 6: Standing
- I can stand as long as I want without extra pain
- I can stand as long as I want but it gives me extra pain
- Pain prevents me from standing for more than 1 hour
- Pain prevents me from standing for more than 30 minutes
- Pain prevents me from standing for more than 10 minutes
- Pain prevents me from standing at all

Section 7: Sleeping
- My sleep is never disturbed by pain
- My sleep is occasionally disturbed by pain
- Because of pain I have less than 6 hours sleep
- Because of pain I have less than 4 hours sleep
- Because of pain I have less than 2 hours sleep
- Pain prevents me from sleeping at all

Section 8: Sex Life (if applicable)
- My sex life is normal and causes no extra pain
- My sex life is normal but causes some extra pain
- My sex life is nearly normal but is very painful
- My sex life is severely restricted by pain
- My sex life is nearly absent because of pain
- Pain prevents any sex life at all

Section 9: Social Life
- My social life is normal and gives me no extra pain
- My social life is normal but increases the degree of pain
- Pain has no significant effect on my social life apart from limiting my more energetic interests e.g. sport
- Pain has restricted my social life and I do not go out as often
- Pain has restricted my social life to my home
- I have no social life because of pain

Section 10: Traveling
- I can travel anywhere without pain
- I can travel anywhere but it gives me extra pain
- Pain is bad but I manage journeys over two hours
- Pain restricts me to journeys of less than one hour
- Pain restricts me to short necessary journeys under 30 minutes
- Pain prevents me from travelling except to receive treatment

NO-FAULT WITH NO FEAR

NECK PAIN DISABILITY INDEX QUESTIONNAIRE

PLEASE READ: This questionnaire is designed to enable us to understand how much your neck pain has affected your ability to manage your everyday activities. Please answer each section by circling the ONE CHOICE that most applies to you. We realize that you may feel that more than one statement may relate to you, but *PLEASE JUST CIRCLE THE ONE. CHOICE WHICH MOST CLOSELY DESCRIBES YOUR PROBLEM RIGHT NOW.*

SECTION 1 - Pain Intensity

A I have no pain at the moment.
B The pain is very mild at the moment.
C The pain is moderate at the moment.
D The pain is fairly severe at the moment.
E The pain is very severe at the moment.
F The pain is the worst imaginable at the moment.

SECTION 2 - Personal Care (Washing, Dressing, etc.)

A I can look after myself normally without causing extra pain.
B I can look after myself normally, but it causes extra pain.
C It is painful to look after myself and I am slow and careful.
D I need some help, but manage most of my personal care.
E I need help every day in most aspects of self care.
F I do not get dressed, I wash with difficulty and stay in bed.

SECTION 3 - Lifting

A I can lift heavy weights without extra pain.
B I can lift heavy weights, but it gives extra pain.
C Pain prevents me from lifting heavy weights off the floor, but I can manage if they are conveniently positioned, for example, on a table.
D Pain prevents me from lifting heavy weights, but I can manage light to medium weights if they are conveniently positioned.
E I can lift very light weights.
F I cannot lift or carry anything at all.

SECTION 4 - Reading

A I can read as much as I want to with no pain in my neck.
B I can read as much as I want to with slight pain in my neck.
C I can read as much as I want to with moderate pain in my neck.
D I cannot read as much as I want because of moderate pain in my neck.
E I cannot read as much as I want because of severe pain in my neck.
F I cannot read at all.

SECTION 5 - Headaches

A I have no headaches at all.
B I have slight headaches which come infrequently.
C I have moderate headaches which come infrequently.
D I have moderate headaches which come frequently.
E I have severe headaches which come frequently.
F I have headaches almost all the time.

SECTION 6 - Concentration

A I can concentrate fully when I want to with no difficulty.
B I can concentrate fully when I want to with slight difficulty.
C I have a fair degree of difficulty in concentrating when I want to.
D I have a lot of difficulty in concentrating when I want to.
E I have a great deal of difficulty in concentrating when I want to.
F I cannot concentrate at all.

SECTION 7 - Work

A I can do as much work as I want to.
B I can only do my usual work, but no more.
C I can do most of my usual work, but no more.
D I cannot do my usual work.
E I can hardly do any work at all.
F I cannot do any work at all.

SECTION 8 - Driving

A I can drive my car without any neck pain.
B I can drive my car as long as I want with slight pain in my neck.
C I can drive my car as long as I want with moderate pain in my neck.
D I cannot drive my car as long as I want because of moderate pain in my neck.
E I can hardly drive at all because of severe pain in my neck.
F I cannot drive my car at all.

SECTION 9 - Sleeping

A I have no trouble sleeping.
B My sleep is slightly disturbed (less than 1 hour sleepless).
C My sleep is mildly disturbed (1-2 hours sleepless).
D My sleep is moderately disturbed (2-3 hours sleepless).
E My sleep is greatly disturbed (3-5 hours sleepless).
F My sleep is completely disturbed (5-7 hours)

SECTION 10 - Recreation

A I am able to engage in all of my recreational activities with no neck pain at all.
B I am able to engage in all of my recreational activities with some pain in my neck.
C I am able to engage in most, but not all of my recreational activities because of pain in my neck.
D I am able to engage in a few of my recreational activities because of pain in my neck.
E I can hardly do any recreational activities because of pain in my neck.
F I cannot do any recreational activities at all.

COMMENTS: _____

NAME: _____ DATE: _____ SCORE: _____

SCORING TECHNIQUE FOR THE OSWESTRY LOW BACK DISABILITY QUESTIONNAIRE AND NECK DISABILITY INDEX

1. Each of the 10 sections is scored separately (0 to 5 points each) and then added up (max. total = 50).

EXAMPLE:

Section 1. Pain Intensity

		Point Value
A. _____	I have no pain at the moment	0
B. _____	The pain is very mild at the moment	1
C. _____	The pain is moderate at the moment	2
D. _____	The pain is fairly severe at the moment	3
E. _____	The pain is very severe at the moment	4
F. _____	The pain is the worst imaginable	5

2. If all 10 sections are completed, simply double the patients score.
3. If a section is omitted, divide the patient's total score by the number of sections completed times 5.

FORMULA: $\frac{\text{PATIENT'S SCORE}}{\text{\# OF SECTIONS COMPLETED X 5}}$ X 100 = _____ % DISABILITY

EXAMPLE:

If 9 of 10 sections are completed, divide the patient's score by 9 X 5 = 45; if........
    Patient's Score: 22
    Number of sections completed: 9 (9 X 5 = 45)
                                 22/45 X 100 = 48 % disability

4. Interpretation of disability scores (from original article):

SCORE	INTERPRETATION OF THE OSWESTRY LBP DISABILITY QUESTIONNAIRE
0-20% Minimal Disability	Can cope w/ most ADL's. Usually no treatment needed, apart from advice on lifting, sitting, posture, physical fitness and diet. In this group, some patients have particular difficulty with sitting and this may be important if their occupation is sedentary (typist, driver, etc.)
20-40% Moderate Disability	This group experiences more pain and problems with sitting, lifting and standing. Travel and social life are more difficult and they may well be off work. Personal care, sexual activity and sleeping are not grossly affected, and the back condition can usually be managed by conservative means.
40-60% Severe Disability	Pain remains the main problem in this group of patients by travel, personal care, social life, sexual activity and sleep are also affected. These patients require detailed investigation.
60-80% Crippled	Back pain impinges on all aspects of these patients' lives both at home and at work. *Positive intervention is required.*
80-100%	These patients are either bed-bound or exaggerating their symptoms. This can be evaluated by careful observation of the patient during the medical examination.

Reference: Fairbanks CT, Couper C, Davies JB, O'Brien JP. The Oswestry low back pain disability questionnaire. Physio Ther 1980;66:271-273.

The Roland-Morris Disability Questionnaire

When your back hurts, you may find it difficult to do some of the things you normally do.

This list contains sentences that people have used to describe themselves when they have back pain. When you read them, you may find that some stand out because they describe you *today*.

As you read the list, think of yourself *today*. When you read a sentence that describes you today, put a tick against it. If the sentence does not describe you, then leave the space blank and go on to the next one. Remember, only tick the sentence if you are sure it describes you today.

1. I stay at home most of the time because of my back.

2. I change position frequently to try and get my back comfortable.

3. I walk more slowly than usual because of my back.

4. Because of my back I am not doing any of the jobs that I usually do around the house.

5. Because of my back, I use a handrail to get upstairs.

6. Because of my back, I lie down to rest more often.

7. Because of my back, I have to hold on to something to get out of an easy chair.

8. Because of my back, I try to get other people to do things for me.

9. I get dressed more slowly then usual because of my back.

10. I only stand for short periods of time because of my back.

11. Because of my back, I try not to bend or kneel down.

12. I find it difficult to get out of a chair because of my back.

13. My back is painful almost all the time.

14. I find it difficult to turn over in bed because of my back.

15. My appetite is not very good because of my back pain.

16. I have trouble putting on my socks (or stockings) because of the pain in my back.

17. I only walk short distances because of my back.

18. I sleep less well because of my back.

19. Because of my back pain, I get dressed with help from someone else.

20. I sit down for most of the day because of my back.

21. I avoid heavy jobs around the house because of my back.

22. Because of my back pain, I am more irritable and bad tempered with people than usual.

23. Because of my back, I go upstairs more slowly than usual.

24. I stay in bed most of the time because of my back.

Note to users:

This questionnaire is taken from: Roland MO, Morris RW. A study of the natural history of back pain. Part 1: Development of a reliable and sensitive measure of disability in low back pain. Spine 1983; 8: 141-144

The score of the RDQ is the total number of items checked – i.e. from a minimum of 0 to a maximum of 24.

It is acceptable to add boxes to indicate where patients should tick each item.

The questionnaire may be adapted for use on-line or by telephone.

NO-FAULT WITH NO FEAR

NO-FAULT WITH NO FEAR

APPENDIX C—NO-FAULT FORMS

NEW YORK MOTOR VEHICLE NO-FAULT INSURANCE LAW
VERIFICATION OF TREATMENT BY ATTENDING PHYSICIAN OR OTHER PROVIDER OF HEALTH SERVICE
(This form is *not* for verification of hospital treatment)

NAME AND ADDRESS OF INSURER OR SELF-INSURER*		NAME, ADDRESS, AND PHONE NUMBER OF INSURER'S CLAIMS REPRESENTATIVE*	
DATE	POLICYHOLDER	POLICY NUMBER	DATE OF ACCIDENT	CLAIM NUMBER

PROVIDER'S NAME AND ADDRESS*

KINDLY COMPLETE AND SUBMIT THIS FORM AS SOON AS POSSIBLE. PLEASE NOTE, THIS COMPLETED FORM MUST BE SUBMITTED TO THE INSURER AS SOON AS REASONABLY POSSIBLE <u>BUT NO LATER THAN 45 DAYS OR 180 DAYS AFTER THE TREATMENT DATE, DEPENDING UPON THE POLICY ENDORSEMENT IN EFFECT AT THE TIME OF THE ACCIDENT</u>. IF YOU ARE UNSURE OF THE APPLICABLE TIME REQUIREMENT, KINDLY CONTACT THE CLAIMS REPRESENTATIVE TO DETERMINE WHICH DEADLINE IS APPLICABLE TO THIS CLAIM.

IF YOU HAVE PREVIOUSLY SUBMITTED AN EARLIER REPORT ON THIS ACCIDENT, YOU NEED ONLY NOTE ANY CHANGES FROM THE INFORMATION PREVIOUSLY FURNISHED AND ADDITIONAL CHARGES.

1. PATIENT'S NAME AND ADDRESS

2. DATE OF BIRTH 3. SEX 4. OCCUPATION (IF KNOWN)

5. DIAGNOSIS AND CONCURRENT CONDITIONS

6. WHEN DID SYMPTOMS FIRST APPEAR? DATE: 7. WHEN DID PATIENT FIRST CONSULT YOU FOR THIS CONDITION? DATE:

8. HAS PATIENT EVER HAD SAME OR SIMILAR CONDITION?
   YES ☐   NO ☐   IF YES, state when and describe:

9. IS CONDITION SOLELY A RESULT OF THIS AUTOMOBILE ACCIDENT?
   YES ☐   NO ☐   IF "NO", explain:

10. IS CONDITION DUE TO INJURY ARISING OUT OF PATIENT'S EMPLOYMENT?
    YES ☐   NO ☐

11. WILL INJURY RESULT IN SIGNIFICANT DISFIGUREMENT OR PERMANENT DISABILITY?
    YES ☐   NO ☐   NOT DETERMINABLE AT THIS TIME ☐
    IF "YES", describe:

12. PATIENT WAS DISABLED (UNABLE TO WORK)
    FROM: _____ THROUGH: _____

13. IF STILL DISABLED THE PATIENT SHOULD BE ABLE TO RETURN TO WORK ON:
    _____ (DATE)

CONTINUE ON PAGE 2

NYS FORM NF-3 (Rev 1/2004)
Page 1 of 3

NO-FAULT WITH NO FEAR

VERIFICATION OF TREATMENT BY ATTENDING PHYSICIAN OR OTHER PROVIDER OF HEALTH SERVICE
PAGE 2

14. WILL THE PATIENT REQUIRE REHABILITATION AND/OR OCCUPATIONAL THERAPY AS A RESULT OF THE INJURIES SUSTAINED IN THIS ACCIDENT?
    YES [ ]   NO [ ]   IF YES, describe your recommendation below:

15. REPORT OF SERVICES RENDERED -- ATTACH ADDITIONAL SHEETS IF NECESSARY

DATE OF SERVICE	PLACE OF SERVICE INCLUDING ZIP CODE	DESCRIPTION OF TREATMENT OR HEALTH SERVICE RENDERED	FEE SCHEDULE TREATMENT CODE	CHARGES
			TOTAL CHARGES TO DATE $	

16. IF TREATING PROVIDER IS DIFFERENT THAN BILLING PROVIDER COMPLETE THE FOLLOWING:

TREATING PROVIDER'S NAME	TITLE	LICENSE OR CERTIFICATION NO.	BUSINESS RELATIONSHIP CHECK APPLICABLE BOX		
			EMPLOYEE	INDEPENDENT CONTRACTOR	OTHER (SPECIFY)

17. IF THE PROVIDER OF SERVICE IS A PROFESSIONAL SERVICE CORPORATION OR DOING BUSINESS UNDER AN ASSUMED NAME (DBA), LIST THE OWNER AND PROFESSIONAL LICENSING CREDENTIALS OF ALL OWNERS (Provide an additional attachment if necessary).

18. IS PATIENT STILL UNDER YOUR CARE FOR THIS CONDITION?   YES [ ]   NO [ ]

19. ESTIMATED DURATION OF FUTURE TREATMENT

PATIENT: Your health provider may agree to accept payment for health services performed directly from your insurer (**Authorization to Pay Benefits**) so that you are not required to make payment to the health provider at the time of service. Such agreement is optional on the part of the health provider and must be signed by both patient and health provider. You may use the optional authorization language provided below, by checking off the designated spot in item 20 of this form.

20. _____ (IF YOU HAVE CHOSEN TO AUTHORIZE THE DIRECT PAYMENT OF BENEFITS BY CHECKING THIS OPTION, **YOU MAY NOT ALSO ENTER INTO AN ASSIGNMENT OF BENEFITS CONTAINED IN #21)**

AUTHORIZATION TO PAY BENEFITS:
I AUTHORIZE PAYMENT OF HEALTH BENEFITS TO THE UNDERSIGNED HEALTH CARE PROVIDER OR SUPPLIER OF SERVICES DESCRIBED BELOW. I RETAIN ALL RIGHTS, PRIVILEGES AND REMEDIES TO WHICH I AM ENTITLED UNDER ARTICLE 51 (THE NO-FAULT PROVISION) OF THE INSURANCE LAW.

PRINT NAME _____   SIGNED _____
                    PATIENT   PATIENT   DATE

CONTINUE ON PAGE 3

NYS FORM NF-3 (Rev 1/2004)
Page 2 of 3

NO-FAULT WITH NO FEAR

VERIFICATION OF TREATMENT BY ATTENDING PHYSICIAN OR OTHER PROVIDER OF HEALTH SERVICE
PAGE 3

PATIENT: Your health provider may agree to have you assign your right to No-Fault benefits from your insurer directly to your health provider (Assignment of Benefits). If you and your health provider agree to an assignment of benefits, you must both sign the agreement contained in # 21 or the prescribed NF-AOB form or its equivalent. The language contained in the assignment of benefits is mandatory and may not be altered or avoided by any other language added to this agreement or other written agreement.

21. _____ (IF YOU HAVE CHOSEN TO ASSIGN YOUR BENEFITS TO THE HEALTH PROVIDER BY CHECKING THIS OPTION, YOU MAY NOT ALSO ENTER INTO AN AUTHORIZATION TO PAY BENEFITS CONTAINED IN ITEM #20 ABOVE)

ASSIGNMENT OF NO-FAULT BENEFITS:
I HEREBY ASSIGN TO THE HEALTH CARE PROVIDER INDICATED BELOW ALL RIGHTS, PRIVILEGES AND REMEDIES TO PAYMENT FOR HEALTH CARE SERVICES PROVIDED BY THE ASSIGNEE TO WHICH I AM ENTITLED UNDER ARTICLE 51 (THE NO-FAULT STATUTE) OF THE INSURANCE LAW. THE ASSIGNEE HEREBY CERTIFIES THAT THEY HAVE NOT RECEIVED ANY PAYMENT FROM OR ON BEHALF OF THE ASSIGNOR AND SHALL NOT PURSUE PAYMENT DIRECTLY FROM THE ASSIGNOR FOR SERVICES PROVIDED BY SAID ASSIGNEE FOR INJURIES SUSTAINED DUE TO THE MOTOR VEHICLE ACCIDENT, NOTWITHSTANDING ANY OTHER AGREEMENT TO THE CONTRARY. THIS AGREEMENT MAY BE REVOKED BY THE ASSIGNEE WHEN BENEFITS ARE NOT PAYABLE BASED UPON THE ASSIGNOR'S LACK OF COVERAGE AND/OR VIOLATION OF A POLICY CONDITION DUE TO THE ACTIONS OR CONDUCT OF THE ASSIGNOR

PRINT NAME _____ SIGNED _____
PATIENT (Assignor)   PATIENT   DATE

PRINT NAME _____ SIGNED _____
PROVIDER OF HEALTH CARE SERVICE (Assignee)   PROVIDER OF HEALTH CARE SERVICE DATE

HAS AN ORIGINAL AUTHORIZATION OR ASSIGNMENT PREVIOUSLY BEEN EXECUTED?   [ ] YES   [ ] NO

IS THE ORIGINAL SIGNATURE OF THE PARTIES ON FILE?   [ ] YES   [ ] NO

ANY PERSON WHO KNOWINGLY AND WITH INTENT TO DEFRAUD ANY INSURANCE COMPANY OR OTHER PERSON FILES AN APPLICATION FOR COMMERCIAL INSURANCE OR A STATEMENT OF CLAIM FOR ANY COMMERCIAL OR PERSONAL INSURANCE BENEFITS CONTAINING ANY MATERIALLY FALSE INFORMATION, OR CONCEALS FOR THE PURPOSE OF MISLEADING, INFORMATION CONCERNING ANY FACT MATERIAL THERETO, AND ANY PERSON WHO, IN CONNECTION WITH SUCH APPLICATION OR CLAIM, KNOWINGLY MAKES OR KNOWINGLY ASSISTS, ABETS, SOLICITS OR CONSPIRES WITH ANOTHER TO MAKE A FALSE REPORT OF THE THEFT, DESTRUCTION, DAMAGE OR CONVERSION OF ANY MOTOR VEHICLE TO A LAW ENFORCEMENT AGENCY, THE DEPARTMENT OF MOTOR VEHICLES OR AN INSURANCE COMPANY, COMMITS A FRAUDULENT INSURANCE ACT, WHICH IS A CRIME, AND SHALL ALSO BE SUBJECT TO A CIVIL PENALTY NOT TO EXCEED FIVE THOUSAND DOLLARS AND THE VALUE OF THE SUBJECT MOTOR VEHICLE OR STATED CLAIM FOR EACH VIOLATION.

DATE	PROVIDER'S SIGNATURE	IRS/TIN IDENTIFICATION NO.	WCB RATING CODE IF NONE, SPECIALTY

*LANGUAGE TO BE FILLED IN BY INSURER OR SELF-INSURER.
NYS FORM NF-3 (Rev 1/2004)
Page 3 of 3

NO-FAULT WITH NO FEAR

NEW YORK MOTOR VEHICLE NO-FAULT INSURANCE LAW
APPLICATION FOR MOTOR VEHICLE NO-FAULT BENEFITS

NAME AND ADDRESS OF INSURER*	NAME, ADDRESS, AND PHONE NUMBER OF INSURER'S CLAIMS REPRESENTATIVE*

DATE	POLICYHOLDER	POLICY NUMBER	DATE OF ACCIDENT	CLAIM NUMBER

TO ENABLE US TO DETERMINE IF YOUR ARE ENTITLED TO BENEFITS UNDER THE NEW YORK NO-FAULT LAW, PLEASE COMPLETE THIS FORM AND RETURN IT PROMPTLY.

IMPORTANT:
1. TO BE ELIGIBLE FOR BENEFITS YOU MUST COMPLETE AND SIGN THIS APPLICATION.
2. YOU MUST SIGN ANY ATTACHED AUTHORIZATION(S).
3. RETURN PROMPTLY WITH COPIES OF ANY BILLS YOU HAVE RECEIVED TO DATE.

NAME AND ADDRESS OF APPLICANT*

1. YOUR NAME	2. PHONE NOS. HOME	BUSINESS

3. YOUR ADDRESS (NO., STREET, CITY OR TOWN AND ZIP CODE)	4. DATE OF BIRTH	5. SOCIAL SECURITY NO.

6. DATE AND TIME OF ACCIDENT A.M. P.M.	7. PLACE OF ACCIDENT (STREET), CITY OR TOWN AND STATE

8. BRIEF DESCRIPTION OF ACCIDENT:

9. DESCRIBE YOUR INJURY:

10. IDENTITY OF VEHICLE YOU OCCUPIED OR OPERATED AT THE TIME OF THE ACCIDENT:

OWNER'S NAME   MAKE   YEAR

THIS VEHICLE WAS: [ ] A BUS OR SCHOOL BUS, OR A MOTORCYCLE   [ ] A TRUCK,   [ ] AN AUTOMOBILE.

	YES	NO
11. WERE YOU THE DRIVER OF THE MOTOR VEHICLE?		
WERE YOU A PASSENGER IN THE MOTOR VEHICLE?		
WERE YOU A PEDESTRIAN?		
WERE YOU A MEMBER OF OUR POLICYHOLDER'S HOUSEHOLD?		
DO YOU OR A RELATIVE WITH WHOM YOU RESIDE OWN A MOTOR VEHICLE?		

CONTINUATION ON NEXT PAGE

NYS FORM NF-2 (Rev 1/2004)
Page 1 of 3

NO-FAULT WITH NO FEAR

APPLICATION FOR MOTOR VEHICLE NO-FAULT BENEFITS - - PAGE TWO

12. WERE YOU TREATED BY A DOCTOR(S) OR OTHER PERSON(S) FURNISHING HEALTH SERVICES?

YES ☐ NO ☐

IF YES, NAME AND ADDRESS OF SUCH DOCTOR(S) OR PERSON(S):

13. IF YOUR WERE TREATED AT A HOSPITAL(S), WERE YOU AN

OUT-PATIENT? ☐ IN-PATIENT? ☐

DATE OF ADMISSION:

HOSPITAL'S NAME AND ADDRESS:

14. AMOUNT OF HEALTH BILLS TO DATE: $	15. WILL YOU HAVE MORE HEALTH TREATMENT(S)? YES ☐ NO ☐	16. AT THE TIME OF YOUR ACCIDENT WERE YOU IN THE COURSE OF YOUR EMPLOYMENT? YES ☐ NO ☐
17. DID YOU LOSE TIME FROM WORK? YES ☐ NO ☐	DATE ABSENCE FROM WORK BEGAN:	HAVE YOU RETURNED TO WORK? YES ☐ NO ☐
IF YES, DATE RETURNED TO WORK:		AMOUNT OF TIME LOST FROM WORK:
18. WHAT ARE YOUR AVERAGE WEEKLY EARNINGS?	NUMBER OF DAYS YOU WORK PER WEEK:	NUMBER OF HOURS YOU WORK PER DAY:

19. WERE YOU RECEIVING UNEMPLOYMENT BENEFITS AT THE TIME OF THE ACCIDENT?

YES ☐ NO ☐

20. LIST NAMES AND ADDRESS OF YOUR EMPLOYER AND OTHER EMPLOYERS FOR ONE YEAR PRIOR TO ACCIDENT DATE AND GIVE OCCUPATION AND DATES OF EMPLOYMENT:

EMPLOYER AND ADDRESS	OCCUPATION	FROM	TO
EMPLOYER AND ADDRESS	OCCUPATION	FROM	TO
EMPLOYER AND ADDRESS	OCCUPATION	FROM	TO

21. AS A RESULT OF YOUR INJURY HAVE YOU HAD ANY OTHER EXPENSES?

YES ☐ NO ☐

IF YES, ATTACH EXPLANATION AND AMOUNTS OF SUCH EXPENSES

22. DUE TO THIS ACCIDENT HAVE YOU RECEIVED OR ARE YOU ELIGIBLE FOR PAYMENTS UNDER ANY OF THE FOLLOWING:

YES ☐ NO ☐

NEW YORK STATE DISABILITY? ☐ ☐

WORKERS' COMPENSATION? ☐ ☐

CONTINUATION ON NEXT PAGE

NYS FORM NF-2 (Rev 1/2004)

NO-FAULT WITH NO FEAR

APPLICATION FOR MOTOR VEHICLE NO-FAULT BENEFITS - - PAGE THREE

THE APPLICANT AUTHORIZES THE INSURER TO SUBMIT ANY AND ALL OF THESE FORMS TO ANOTHER PARTY OR INSURER IF SUCH IS NECESSARY TO PERFECT ITS RIGHTS OF RECOVERY PROVIDED FOR UNDER THE NO-FAULT LAW.

THIS FORM IS SUBSCRIBED AND AFFIRMED BY THE
APPLICANT AS TRUE UNDER THE PENALTIES OF PERJURY

ANY PERSON WHO KNOWINGLY AND WITH INTENT TO DEFRAUD ANY INSURANCE COMPANY OR OTHER PERSON FILES AN APPLICATION FOR COMMERCIAL INSURANCE OR A STATEMENT OF CLAIM FOR ANY COMMERCIAL OR PERSONAL INSURANCE BENEFITS CONTAINING ANY MATERIALLY FALSE INFORMATION, OR CONCEALS FOR THE PURPOSE OF MISLEADING, INFORMATION CONCERNING ANY FACT MATERIAL THERETO, AND ANY PERSON WHO, IN CONNECTION WITH SUCH APPLICATION OR CLAIM, KNOWINGLY MAKES OR KNOWINGLY ASSISTS, ABETS, SOLICITS OR CONSPIRES WITH ANOTHER TO MAKE A FALSE REPORT OF THE THEFT, DESTRUCTION, DAMAGE OR CONVERSION OF ANY MOTOR VEHICLE TO A LAW ENFORCEMENT AGENCY, THE DEPARTMENT OF MOTOR VEHICLES OR AN INSURANCE COMPANY, COMMITS A FRAUDULENT INSURANCE ACT, WHICH IS A CRIME, AND SHALL ALSO BE SUBJECT TO A CIVIL PENALTY NOT TO EXCEED FIVE THOUSAND DOLLARS AND THE VALUE OF THE SUBJECT MOTOR VEHICLE OR STATED CLAIM FOR EACH VIOLATION.

_____ _____
SIGNATURE   DATE

DO NOT DETACH
AUTHORIZATION FOR RELEASE OF WORK AND OTHER LOSS INFORMATION

THIS AUTHORIZATION OR PHOTOCOPY THEREOF, WILL AUTHORIZE YOU TO FURNISH ALL INFORMATION YOU MAY HAVE REGARDING MY WAGES, SALARY OR OTHER LOSS WHILE EMPLOYED BY YOU. YOUR ARE AUTHORIZED TO PROVIDE THIS INFORMATION IN ACCORDANCE WITH THE NEW YORK COMPREHENSIVE MOTOR VEHICLE INSURANCE REPARATIONS ACT (NO-FAULT LAW).

_____ _____
NAME (PRINT OR TYPE)   SOCIAL SECURITY NO.

_____ _____
SIGNATURE   DATE

DO NOT DETACH
AUTHORIZATION FOR RELEASE OF HEALTH SERVICE OR TREATMENT INFORMATION

THIS AUTHORIZATION OR PHOTOCOPY THEREOF, WILL AUTHORIZE YOU TO FURNISH ALL INFORMATION YOU MAY HAVE REGARDING MY CONDITION WHILE UNDER YOUR OBSERVATION OR TREATMENT, INCLUDING THE HISTORY OBTAINED, X-RAYS AND PHYSICAL FINDINGS, DIAGNOSIS AND PROGNOSIS. YOU ARE AUTHORIZED TO PROVIDE THIS INFORMATION IN ACCORDANCE WITH THE NEW YORK COMPREHENSIVE MOTOR VEHICLE INSURANCE REPARATIONS ACT (NO-FAULT LAW).

_____
NAME (PRINT OR TYPE)

_____ _____
SIGNATURE   DATE

(IF THE APPLICANT IS A MINOR, PARENT OR GUARDIAN SHALL SIGN AND INDICATE CAPACITY AND RELATIONSHIP).

*LANGUAGE TO BE FILLED IN BY INSURER OR SELF-INSURER.
NYS FORM NF-2 (Rev 1/2004)
Page 3 of 3

NO-FAULT WITH NO FEAR

NEW YORK MOTOR VEHICLE NO-FAULT INSURANCE LAW
ASSIGNMENT OF BENEFITS FORM

(FOR ACCIDENTS OCCURRING ON AND AFTER 3/1/02)

I, _____ ("Assignor") hereby assign to Assignee") _____
   (Print patient's name)(Print hospital or health care provider name)
all rights privileges and remedies to payment for health care services provided by assignee to which I am entitled under Article 51 (the No-Fault statute) of the Insurance Law.

The Assignee hereby certifies that they have not received any payment from or on behalf of the Assignor and shall not pursue payment directly from the Assignor for services provided by said Assignee for injuries sustained due to the motor vehicle accident which occurred on, _____ not withstanding any other agreement to the contrary.
                                                                    (Print accident date)

This agreement may be revoked by the assignee when benefits are not payable based upon the assignor's lack of coverage and/or violation of a policy condition due to the actions or conduct of the assignor.

ANY PERSON WHO KNOWINGLY AND WITH INTENT TO DEFRAUD ANY INSURANCE COMPANY OR OTHER PERSON FILES AN APPLICATION FOR COMMERCIAL INSURANCE OR A STATEMENT OF CLAIM FOR ANY COMMERCIAL OR PERSONAL INSURANCE BENEFITS CONTAINING ANY MATERIALLY FALSE INFORMATION, OR CONCEALS FOR THE PURPOSE OF MISLEADING, INFORMATION CONCERNING ANY FACT MATERIAL THERETO, AND ANY PERSON WHO, IN CONNECTION WITH SUCH APPLICATION OR CLAIM, KNOWINGLY MAKES OR KNOWINGLY ASSISTS, ABETS, SOLICITS OR CONSPIRES WITH ANOTHER TO MAKE A FALSE REPORT OF THE THEFT, DESTRUCTION, DAMAGE OR CONVERSION OF ANY MOTOR VEHICLE TO A LAW ENFORCEMENT AGENCY, THE DEPARTMENT OF MOTOR VEHICLES OR AN INSURANCE COMPANY, COMMITS A FRAUDULENT INSURANCE ACT, WHICH IS A CRIME, AND SHALL ALSO BE SUBJECT TO A CIVIL PENALTY NOT TO EXCEED FIVE THOUSAND DOLLARS AND THE VALUE OF THE SUBJECT MOTOR VEHICLE OR STATED CLAIM FOR EACH VIOLATION.

_____   _____
(Print name of Patient)   (Signature of Patient)

_____   _____
                                  (Date of signature)

_____
(Address of Patient)

_____   _____
(Print name of Provider)   (Signature of Provider)

_____   _____
                                  (Date of signature)

_____
(Address of Provider)

NYS FORM NF-AOB (Rev 1/2004)

NO-FAULT WITH NO FEAR

APPENDIX D

COMMONLY USED ICD-10 DIAGNOSIS CODES BY CHIROPRACTORS IN THE NO-FAULT CLINIC

Cervical

S13.4XXA	Sprain of ligaments of cervical spine, initial encounter
S14.2XXA	Injury of nerve root of cervical spine, initial encounter
S14.3XXA	Injury of brachial plexus, initial encounter
S16.1XXA	Strain of muscle, fascia and tendon at neck level, initial encounter
M99.01	Segmental and somatic dysfunction of cervical region
M99.11	Subluxation complex (vertebral) of cervical region
M25.50	Pain in unspecified joint (Cervical facet)
M54.2	Cervicalgia
M54.12	Radiculopathy, cervical region
M47.811	Spondylosis without myelopathy or radiculopathy, occipito-atlanto-axial region
M47.812	Spondylosis without myelopathy or radiculopathy, cervical region
M47.21	Other spondylosis with radiculopathy, occipito-atlanto-axial region
M47.22	Other spondylosis with radiculopathy, cervical region
M47.23	Other spondylosis with radiculopathy, cervicothoracic region
M47.892	Other spondylosis, cervical region

M47.893	Other spondylosis, cervicothoracic
M50.11	Cervical disc disorder with radiculopathy, occipito-atlanto-axial region
M50.12	Cervical disc disorder with radiculopathy, mid-cervical region
M50.13	Cervical disc disorder with radiculopathy, cervicothoracic region

Thoracic

S23.3XXA	Sprain of ligaments of thoracic spine, initial encounter
S24.2XXA	Injury of nerve root of thoracic spine, initial encounter
M99.02	Segmental and somatic dysfunction of thoracic region
M99.12	Subluxation complex (vertebral) of thoracic region
M25.50	Pain in unspecified joint (Thoracic facet)
M54.6	Pain in thoracic spine
M54.14	Radiculopathy, thoracic region
M51.14	Intervertebral disc disorders with radiculopathy, thoracic region
M51.15	Intervertebral disc disorders with radiculopathy, thoracolumbar region
M47.814	Spondylosis without myelopathy or radiculopathy, thoracic region
M47.815	Spondylosis without myelopathy or radiculopathy, thoracolumbar region
M47.24	Other spondylosis with radiculopathy, thoracic region

M47.25	Other spondylosis with radiculopathy, thoracolumbar region
M47.894	Other spondylosis, thoracic region
M47.895	Other spondylosis, thoracolumbar region

Lumbar

S33.8XXA	Sprain of other parts of lumbar spine and pelvis, initial encounter
S39.012A	Strain of muscle, fascia and tendon of lower back
M54.5	Low Back Pain
M54.16	Radiculopathy, lumbar region
M54.17	Radiculopathy, lumbosacral region
M51.16	Intervertebral disc disorders with radiculopathy, lumbar region
M54.31	Sciatica, right side
M54.32	Sciatica, left side
M47.816	Spondylosis without myelopathy or radiculopathy, lumbar region
M47.26	Other spondylosis with radiculopathy, lumbar region
M47.896	Other spondylosis, lumbar region

Pelvic

M99.04	Segmental and somatic dysfunction of sacral region
M99.05	Segmental and somatic dysfunction of pelvic region
M99.14	Subluxation complex (vertebral) of sacral region
M99.15	Subluxation complex (vertebral) of pelvic region

M25.50	Pain in unspecified joint (Sacroiliac joint)
M54.5	Low Back Pain (Sacroiliac joint)
M54.17	Radiculopathy, lumbosacral region
M47.817	Spondylosis without myelopathy or radiculopathy, lumbosacral region
M51.17	Intervertebral disc disorders with radiculopathy, lumbosacral region
M25.50	Pain in unspecified joint (Sacroiliac joint)

Other

F07.81	Postconcussion syndrome
G44.309	Post-traumatic headache, not intractable, unspecified
G44.209	Tension-type headache, not intractable, unspecified
M62.81	Muscle weakness (generalized)
M62.830	Muscle spasm of back
M62.831	Muscle spasm of calf
M62.838	Other muscle spasm
R26.81	Unsteadiness on feet
R29.2	Abnormal reflex
R29.3	Abnormal posture
R60.0	Localized edema
G89.11	Acute pain due to trauma
G89.21	Chronic pain due to trauma

NOTE REGARDING EXTENSIONS A, D, AND S:

The extension "A" (as in S13.4XXA) for initial encounter is to be used for all ACTIVE CARE visits- not just the first visit.

The extension "D" for subsequent encounters is the visit(s) after the active phase of treatment terminates. For instance, if a medical provider refers a patient to a chiropractor for care, once care is completed with the chiropractor and the patient is being followed up with by the medical provider, that constitutes the subsequent encounter.

The extension "S" is for sequelae- Sequelae refers to the

complications or conditions that arise as a direct result of an injury (residual effects). These residual effects can be pain, scar tissue, loss of range of motion, etc.

Generally, a **sequelae code** such as **S13.4XXS** is coded secondary to the sequelae itself. For instance, residual pain in the cervical spine following a sprain would be coded in the following manner:

S13.4XXA	Sprain of ligaments of cervical spine
M54.2	Cervical pain (as primary symptom)
S13.4XXS	This indicates this pain is a **sequelae** of a cervical Sprain.

(FROM: Coding for Strains and Sprains in ICD-10, *Dynamic Chiropractic – June 1, 2015, Vol. 33, Issue 1)*

ABOUT THE AUTHOR

A graduate of New York Chiropractic College, Dr. S. Joseph Metz has been practicing chiropractic in New York for nearly twenty-five years. In addition to a 14-year private practice, he has worked extensively in many of the metropolitan area's so-called "no-fault" clinics, which almost exclusively serve patients who have been injured in motor vehicle accidents. Dr. Metz is also certified in electromyography, and has traveled throughout the United States performing electrodiagnostic testing in offices around the country. He is an avid runner, and lives, runs, and writes in New York.

www.ingramcontent.com/pod-product-compliance
Lightning Source LLC
Chambersburg PA
CBHW050202230526
45470CB00001B/210